Caring for Yourself While Caring for Others

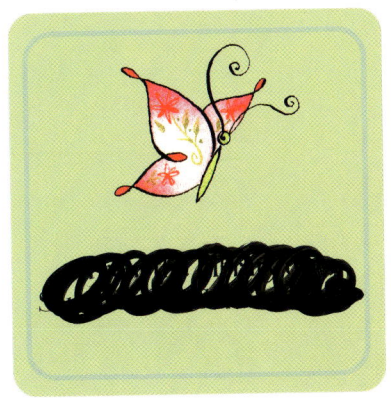

Sandy McClanab

Caring for Yourself While Caring for Others

A Caregiver's Survival and Renewal Guide

Lawrence M. Brammer, Ph.D., and Marian L. Bingea, M.A.

VANTAGE PRESS
New York

Scriptural quotations in this book are from the King James Bible.

FIRST EDITION

All rights reserved, including the right of
reproduction in whole or in part in any form.

Copyright © 1999 by Lawrence M. Brammer, Ph.D.,
and Marian L. Bingea, M.A.

Published by Vantage Press, Inc.
516 West 34th Street, New York, New York 10001

Manufactured in the United States of America
ISBN: 0-533-12876-5

Library of Congress Catalog Card No.: 98-90666

0 9 8 7 6 5 4 3

To the Reverend Doctor Richard J. Bingea (1920–96). We honor his many years of service to countless people of all ages as a pastor and ecumenical religious leader. He was the consummate caregiver, sensitive, loving, caring, and compassionate to all with whom he came in contact—especially to his family, friends, parishioners, and those hurting in body, mind, and spirit.

Contents

Foreword	xi
Introduction: Why Read This Book?	xiii
Part I: Coping and Survival	**1**
1. Unsung Heroes	3
You as Caregiver	3
What Is Self-Care?	7
Caregiver Burnout	9
Becoming a Survivor	13
Caregivers Who Function Optimally	15
Varieties of Care	17
Multicultural Caregiving Perspectives	21
A Rosier Future in Sight	24
Notes	25
Recommended Reading	26
2. Survival of the Fittest	27
Caregivers as Skilled Copers	27
Potential Danger–Fight or Flight?	30
Building and Using Support	31
Coping with Hassles and Stressors	35
Changing Negative Thoughts	42
Welcome to the Hardiness Hall of Fame	47
Notes	47
Recommended Reading	48

Part II: Knowing Your Inner Resources   49

3. Knowing Your Inner Strengths   51

    Spiritual Resources   51
    Meaning in Spirituality   53
    Morals and Ethics   55
    Belonging to a Community   57
    Values   58
    Beliefs   62
    Your Sense of Humor   62
    Your Inner Journey   67
    Notes   67

4. The Quest for Intimacy   68

    When Intimacy Fades   68
    What Are Your Choices?   71
    A Final Word   78
    Notes   79
    Recommended Reading   79

5. How to Make Your Life Easier   80

    Problem Solving   80
    Trial and Error   81
    Logical Problem Solving   82
    Intuitive and Creative Styles of Problem Solving   86
    Experiential Focusing   89
    Communication Effectiveness   93
    So, You Can Make Your Life Easier   105
    Notes   106
    Recommended Reading   106

Part III: Facing Difficult Feelings — 107

6. The Journey through Grief — 109

Grieving — 110
What Makes Mourning Difficult? — 114
Anticipatory and Delayed Grieving — 117
Handling Your Grief — 118
Resources for Grieving — 121
Gender Differences in Grieving — 126
Child Grief — 127
Multicultural Modes of Grieving — 127
Some Final Words — 130
Notes — 130
Recommended Reading — 131

7. Depression: A Problem for Caregivers — 132

What Is Depression? — 132
Inoculating Yourself against Depression — 136
Hope, Hopelessness, and Despair — 138
A Look Back — 143
Notes — 144
Recommended Reading — 144

8. The Triple Tyrannies: Anger, Guilt, and Anxiety — 145

Coping with Your Frustration and Anger — 145
The Ill/Well Spouse — 149
Abusive Behavior — 150
Repeat Caregivers — 151
Forgiveness — 151
Canceling Guilt Trips — 154
A Summary of Guidelines for Managing Guilt — 158
Banning Worry and Panic — 159
The Worrying Caregiver — 160
Summary of Thoughts on the Triple Tyrannies — 164
Notes — 165

Part IV: Knowing Your Community Resources — 167

9. Your External Resources — 169

    Easing the Burden — 169
    Care Managers — 170
    Community Services for Caregivers — 172
    Religious Resources — 178
    Support Services for Caregivers — 180
    Computer Internet — 183
    Networking — 183
    Counseling — 183
    A Last Word on Resources — 186
    Notes — 186
    Recommended Reading — 187

Part V: Planning for Wellness and Renewal — 189

10. Staying Well and Keeping Fit — 191

    Wellness for Caregivers — 191
    Vulnerability to Pain — 198
    Lifestyle Renewal — 201
    Life Review — 208
    Putting It All Together — 210
    Notes — 210
    Recommended References — 211

Appendixes

Appendix A: Making a Self-Care Contract — 215
Appendix B: Internet Web Sites for Caregivers — 217
Appendix C: Caregiver Survey — 221

Foreword

Caring for Yourself While Caring for Others is aimed at one of the most vulnerable populations in America—caregivers themselves. These are the hidden heroines and heroes who often sacrifice their health, and sometimes their lives, while caring for others.

Larry Brammer and Marian Bingea have included the critical issues which face both family and professional caregivers as they provide physical and emotional health and human services to loved ones who are ill and disabled. The information and discussion is current, incisive and comprehensive.

Especially welcome are the sections on spirituality, intimacy, intuitive problem-solving, humor and multicultural implications. There is a multitude of how-to suggestions for knowing oneself, improving communication, overcoming caregiver stress and burnout, and seeking support.

                        Bonnie Genevay, MSW
                        Author, Trainer & Consultant in
                        Gerontology & Bereavement

Introduction: Why Read This Book?

"For better or worse, in sickness and in health," is the passionate vow uttered by wedding couples. However, this passion cannot compare with a caregiver's love and devotion. Unfortunately, this passion is soon replaced by exhaustion, loneliness, and anger. Yet many caregivers deem their labor an expression of love. This love must include self-love also, in the form of self-care.

The focus of this book is your self-care. Personal survival and renewal are themes emphasized throughout, so look on this book as your personal caregiver survival kit. Recent surveys indicate that one in four U.S. households has at least one person as a caregiver for a family member who is fifty or older. If we add the caregivers for younger disabled persons, it would be closer to one in three households that has a primary caregiver. So, even if you are not a caregiver now, considering the increases in longevity and handicapped newborns, it is highly likely that you will, sometime soon, be a caregiver.

We cannot give you a profile of the typical caregiver, but we can convey a compassionate understanding of the burdens you bear, the frustrations, loneliness, and occasional hopelessness you experience. We also recognize that your caregiving provides satisfactions and feelings of accomplishment for this sacred mission.

You must read this book to discover the essentials for achieving your survival and renewal goals. These are essential self-care skills that you learn and apply quickly while reading this book:

1. Prevention and coping with burnout.
2. Building and using support networks.
3. Coping with hassles and stressors.
4. Changing self-defeating thoughts.
5. Strengthening spirituality.
6. Developing a sense of humor.
7. Satisfying needs for intimacy.
8. Coping with depression, despair, grief, anger, guilt, and worry.
9. Building communication skills.
10. Making plans for wellness and renewal.
11. Developing a self-care contract.
12. Planning for life after caregiving.

We have used our extensive scholarship, research, and caregiving experience to write this book. Our personal interviews with twenty current caregivers gave us a wealth of data on how they perceived their caring roles. Where we have used the research of others, we assigned a citation number matched to the notes at the ends of the chapters.

This book is not about techniques for performing your caregiving tasks. There are many printed and community resources to help you provide caregiving activities for various types of disabled people. This book is primarily about you and what you can do to tap your inner emotional and spiritual strengths, as well as to develop useful coping skills and attitudes. Thus, not only is it a survival guide, but we hope it will also be an aid to renewal and enrichment so that your life will continue to have meaning and satisfaction while you are performing your arduous caregiving tasks. To provide these self-help resources, we draw upon the rich traditions of psychology, social work, philosophy, religion, medicine, education, and cross-cultural studies.

Since the focus is on self-care rather than on methods for providing care to another person, references are provided at the end of each chapter for help with specific kinds of care. Professional care managers and long-term care staff members will also find this book useful personally and in staff development.

The backgrounds of the authors include a variety of experiences related to caregiving. Lawrence Brammer, Ph.D. is a retired university professor of counseling psychology who specializes in issues related to aging, helping functions, and coping with life transitions. He has a master's and a Ph.D. from Stanford. Currently he writes, speaks, and consults on a variety of applied psychology topics. He has published six books, seven chapters in books, and over one hundred professional research and conceptual articles. Two of his books, *The Helping Relationship* and *Therapeutic Counseling and Psychotherapy,* are published in sixth and seventh editions, respectively. His general book, *How to Cope with Life Transitions,* is directly relevant to this book. Presently he is teaching disaster courses for the American Red Cross and takes local and national disaster assignments as a volunteer mental health specialist. He serves in the caring ministry program of his local church.

Marian L. Bingea has a master's degree in Scandinavian languages and literature and two bachelor's degrees in history and Scandinavian studies. She is a professional organist who performs regularly. Marian brought up five children and cared for her ailing husband for many years until his recent death. As a pastor's wife, she was deeply involved in caring ministries for three decades. Marian also was employed for several years as a social service worker in a large city-county hospital. Currently she is a volunteer at a local hospice. Thus, she brings a wealth of experience in direct and vicarious caregiving to this book.

We thank the caregivers who, in our interviews with them, freely and courageously shared their personal experiences. We appreciated Marian Brammer's encouragement and support during this project. We acknowledge with thanks the skillful word processing and helpful editorial suggestions of Jordis Young. We also thank Lenore Franzen for her professional editorial suggestions.

      Lawrence M. Brammer, Ph.D.
      Marian L. Bingea, MA
      March 1998

Caring for Yourself While Caring for Others

PART I
Coping and Survival

1
Unsung Heroes

The capacity to care is the thing that gives life its deepest significance.
—Pablo Casals, renowned cellist

You as Caregiver

Battles produce heroes, businesses and sports have their heroes. Even families have unsung heroes—the folk who uncomplainingly, courageously, and tirelessly get the job done. They go way beyond the call of duty. Perhaps you do not think of yourself as doing heroic things, but the caregivers we know deserve hero medals.

Caregivers find themselves thrust into unsung hero roles in two ways. A family member or friend suffers a sudden heart attack, stroke, or accident. You are the most willing and available to resolve the crisis. The other way caregivers acquire their role is when a relative or friend slowly deteriorates with dementia, Parkinson's, or multiple sclerosis, for example. Thus, perhaps willingly at first, you become part of that vast army of invisible and unpaid workers called *caregivers*. It is one job you never apply for.

You are asked to sacrifice your leisure, vacations, privacy, and personal pleasures to care for friends and loved ones. Furthermore, the period of service is undefined and is subject to your stamina and commitment and the course of your patient's illness or recovery. You are, indeed, the unsung heroes. Those of you who are caregivers now appreciate the need for self-care to survive and renew.

Let's listen to a few caregivers. A **single child** caring for aged parents: "I feel so alone doing this work. I wish I had some sibs to share the tasks." A **spouse**: "I feel like a prisoner. He clings to me constantly." A **daughter**: "This is a very painful time, but I see it as a kind of ministry." A **stepchild**: "We have problems sharing the responsibilities. Resentments are beginning to spoil our relationship." **Lesbian and gay** caregivers: "We are hurt by the discrimination and lack of support from family and friends." A **working wife**: "I tried to work and take care of my dad and my family, but it was too much. I crumbled." A **second wife**: "After years of caregiving, I began to wonder if it would ever stop. Now I'm caring for my second husband."

Printed words cannot do justice to a caregiver's intense feelings. While some feel rewarded and fulfilled, we know from our experience, interviews, and research that most of you also feel burdened. Surprise, exasperation, regret, loneliness, fear, panic, guilt, sadness, relief, and privilege are heard frequently. We trust that our discussions of caregiving will enable you to face the challenges, reduce the burdens, and reap the rewards.

As revealed in the introductory caregiver comments, not all caregivers perceive their roles as a severe burden. They are frustrated at times, but some providers consider caregiving a service opportunity, a personal ministry, a labor of love, or an opportunity to receive satisfaction of a "need to be needed." In any case, caregiving, for many who have this positive outlook, adds meaning to life. One of the caregivers in our survey said, for example, that she felt caring for her elderly parent was a special privilege. "I received more than I gave," was her final response.

Long-Distance Caregiving

Since family mobility is so high, today the family member needing care is often in a distant place. So, the primary caregiver must arrange for home care by a professional care manager. This professional care manager hires the caregivers and provides home services. Local area agencies on aging can help arrange inexpensive services. But having professional care for a distant loved one does not diminish your anguish and daily concern about the loved one's welfare.

Grandparents caring for their own or other's grandchildren is a growing enterprise. According to the U.S. Census, about 3.7 million children live in households where neither parent lives and that are headed by grandparents, Many social problems contribute to the 40 percent increase in that situation during the past decade. Grandparents are thrust into a caregiving role just as they retire to enjoy leisure, travel, and financial stability. This new role of caregiving postpones these plans indefinitely, thus contributing to their feelings of anger and grief.[1]

Multiple Caregiving

Perhaps you are a caregiver for more than one person now. This book was written especially for you, in order to ease these multiple burdens. Perhaps you are also a member of the "sandwich generation," raising children while caring for aging parents . . . and being a spouse at the same time. This is a most difficult part to play in life's drama, since it places almost impossible demands on one's time, patience, and energy. These caregivers have been called *middle-aged kin-keepers*.

The realities of multiple responsibilities are illustrated by an example from our study of caregivers for the American Gerontological Society.[2] **Emma**, a sixty-nine-year-old woman, had been caregiving for over forty years with little respite. First, she brought up two children of her own.

Later, her husband of twelve years developed multiple sclerosis and required constant care in the later stages. After his death, she nursed her son with the same disease until he was placed in a nursing home, where he still resides. In the meantime, her long-term boarder became disabled, and she cared for him for twenty years, until he died in a treatment center for alcoholics. Now her ninety-six-year-old mother requires constant attention, broken only by respite provided by a distant brother and sister who only sporadically come to her home.

Emma accepted this responsibility remarkably well, but she confided in the interview, "I have no time for me, to care for me, even to make medical appointments for myself." At this point her tears flowed freely. She indicated that she had not unburdened herself emotionally for years. She was a self-sufficient survivor with many good coping skills. While she told her story stoically, a remarkable cheerfulness seeped through. She also performed her caregiving tasks with apparent efficacy.

While this caregiver's story is quite unusual, it illustrates the need for the caregiver's self-care and support. It emphasized dramatically how emotionally draining continuous and multiple caregiving can be. It also underlines the need to have outlets for emotional relief and sharing the burden with someone the caregiver trusts.

Meaning of Caring

Caring covers many humane actions, including:

- Showing compassion and telling the other person you care.
- Expressing love.
- Being available when you say you will be.

- Showing interest in the other person's welfare with words and deeds.
- Sharing other persons' joy, or being with them in their sorrow.
- Listening even when you want to be talking.
- Hearing and responding with empathy.[3]

Upon reflection, how do you show your caring?

What Is Self-Care?

While caring for others is an admirable and unselfish act, it is often done by neglecting the caregiver's own care. Caring for others adequately requires equal concern for your self-care, especially since you probably are in it for the long haul.

Self-care means loving, honoring, and accepting yourself. It is based on a conviction that you deserve honor and respect for what you are. This self-caring attitude goes beyond keeping fit and managing everyday stressors. It means setting limits to the demands and expectations of caregiving in a way that says, "I'm doing the best I can in this situation; don't push me. Let me decide my limitations."

Responsibility for Self-Care

Each of us is responsible for our own welfare. To do our caregiving responsibly we must put our own care first, so we are capable of doing our best. This focus on self-care is not the extreme self-centeredness that has infected our me-first society. It is not a narcissistic form of self-love or self-esteem that ignores your patient; nor does it represent an arrogant, better-than-thou attitude. Self-care is based upon the idea that you must base your love, respect, and compassion for others on a healthy self-love and self-respect.

What Could Prevent You from Achieving this Self-Love and Respect?

1. *Learned attitudes from our culture, and especially family, are the greatest help or obstacles to developing self-respect.* You learn very early to turn against yourself. Parents make contradictory demands; teachers evaluate you critically; your associates tease and ridicule you. So, under this constant barrage of high expectations and criticisms you tend to perceive yourself as inadequate, unworthy, and undeserving. Since you very likely are a parent also, you know that you cannot blame your parents totally for the presumed idiosyncrasies in your upbringing. As stated previously, you must take the responsibility for your own behavior. We mention these child-rearing consequences only to point out more clearly how the obstacles to effective self-care develop.
2. *As a caregiver you probably do not get the appreciation and gratitude you think you deserve.* Many care recipients are so impaired or so centered on their own needs and pain that they cannot give the appreciation that caregivers would like. You probably labor under feelings of inadequacy at times, and you probably are your most severe critic. Eleanor Roosevelt, the revered wife of Pres. Franklin D. Roosevelt, had some good advice for caregivers: "No one can make you feel inferior without your consent." In other words, we malign ourselves. Are you too hard on yourself?

3. *Another obstacle to self-care is not having a clear idea of who you are and what you want.* This sets you up as an easy target for requests from family or friends. Do you have trouble saying no to friends who try to persuade you to take on more responsibility than you want? They make it difficult by sugar-coating the request, saying that it will take only a few hours; however, they do not tell you that time commitments escalate. When you say yes but really want to say no, your self-loathing later becomes even more pronounced. Is saying no a problem for you?
4. *Finding time for self-care is a problem for caregivers.* If you add self-care to your caregiving time, along with commitments to family, job, and community, you find yourself under an enormous burden. You may say, however, that you are strong and dedicated and that you are a plucky survivor. If so, great, but the price of this sustained energy drain and cumulative care demands is high. It leads to the condition popularly known as "burnout." Some caregivers call it compassion fatigue. Do you find it difficult to take time for yourself? How many of the obstacles to self-care cited here apply to you? What can you do to remove or reduce those obstacles?

Caregiver Burnout

Burnout is a state of total physical and emotional exhaustion. **Georgia**, a homemaker in her midfifties, was a caregiver for thirty years. She also worked part-time outside her home. First, she cared for her grandmother, who had brought her up. (Her father was killed when she was an infant, and her mother worked full-time.) Then Georgia cared for her disabled alcoholic husband for ten years, until she divorced him. As a single parent she cared for her three young children until they were independent. At that time she became the primary caregiver for her elderly stepmother, and she has done this for the past twelve years. Presently her stepmother is barely mobile, has deteriorating vision, and is in constant pain.

Georgia spends thirty-five hours a week taking care of her stepmother and thirty-five hours a week in outside employment. She has not had a vacation for as long as she can remember. Her low family income prevents her from employing respite services, and she has few relatives she can depend upon. Georgia said to the interviewer, "I'm totally burned out," and went on to describe her frustrations, despair, and hopelessness. Her cumulative anger seeped into the conversation frequently. Probably you, too, are wondering how Georgia had the strength and stamina to go on this long.

From Georgia's and other caregivers' experiences we can construct a composite picture of the burned-out caregiver. This condition afflicts especially the most conscientious and hardworking caregivers.

Signs of Burnout

- Exhaustion—physical and emotional—not eased by rest: "I've had it; no more."
- Resentment and open anger at times, but most anger directed at self.
- Feeling overwhelmed by responsibility: "Some days I don't think I can go on."
- Loss of interest in formerly pleasurable activity: "I don't have any fun anymore."
- Digestive problems and loss of appetite: "My body is complaining something fierce."

- Vague aches and pains: "My joints are sure giving me trouble since I took this job."
- Difficulties going to sleep and staying asleep: "I'm using too many tranquilizers."
- Restlessness and irritability: "Some days I just want to junk the whole mess."
- Apathy and denial of feelings: "I just don't care anymore."
- Memory, concentration, and attention problems: "I can't keep my mind on my work."
- Cynicism and hopelessness about caregiving: "What's the use? Everyone has forgotten me. They don't care."

Beware—the deteriorative process in burnout is insidious. You will find that caregivers wear down gradually, in the following stages:

- Disillusionment and frustration with their current caregiving situation.
- Depression and hopelessness about the future, along with severe self-criticism.
- Demoralization and disengagement from caregiving tasks; emotional detachment.
- Dysfunction—total inability to carry out caregiving responsibility; collapse of body systems. The caregiver requires total care.

Coping with Approaching Burnout

All is not lost. There is hope! The following guidelines will be supplemented by additional suggestions later under "Strategies for Stress Management," "Lifestyle Renewal," and "Planning for Wellness and Renewal."

- Give yourself permission to feel what you are experiencing—joy, pain, disappointment, and regret, for example.
- Think of all the strengths you have as a person and as a caregiver—sensitivity, generosity, compassion, and friendliness, for example. This task may be difficult, since it is much easier to list your faults. Start with memories of events during which you felt strong competent, energized, and confident.
- Write your affirmations. For example: "I am competent; I am a worthwhile person; I can do many tasks well." Look at your affirmation strength list every day. Attach it to your mirror and repeat the affirmations as you look at yourself.
- Take personal control of your self-care. Do not leave this critical responsibility to your relatives, pastor, therapist, or support group, who have their own needs and problems. Thus, when *you* take charge of your self-care you will be able to give your care receiver more cheerful and effective care.
- Rehearse how you will say no to requests for taking new responsibilities when you feel you are already overcommitted.
- Think about how you would request other family members to take over when you reach that last stage of burnout.
- Learn to live with detached concern. This means staying emotionally involved with your receiver and at the same time striving for objectivity. This is a difficult balance to achieve, but it is necessary for survival.
- Find the best balance among your commitments to community, family, church, and patient care. Think about using this principle of balance in other domains of your life.

- Set aside your own special time for what you find fulfilling and relaxing. This list is endless and could include reading, walking, playing an instrument, meditating, or knitting. Guard this time zealously against the numerous forces that want to take it.
- From the discussion to follow make a list of survivor behaviors that you wish to acquire.

Becoming a Survivor

Fortunately, we humans are born with strong resistance to stressors. We learn over a lifetime to cope with unjust and distressing situations. Our learned coping skills of support networking, changing thoughts, stress management, and problem solving help us to survive and to avoid labeling ourselves as victims.

Survivors often have suffered from abuse, deception, mistreatment, and violence. Survivors, according to Al Sieberts's research, have come through difficult family upbringing, disasters, holocausts, and accidents, but rebounded with new positive goals and learned important life lessons and were ready to rebuild their lives.[4]

Survivors were able to tap their deepest strengths after the distressful event. Prisoners of war confined for long periods, holocaust victims suffering cruelties for years, and survivors of devastating natural disasters are examples. Positive survival learnings appeared to come out of their struggles—learnings that could not be taught formally. An inspiring example is that of Dr. Victor Frankl, who spent years in a death camp during the Holocaust. His search for meaning in each moment of suffering enabled him to survive and become one of the most productive contributors to psychotherapy in the post–World War II period.[5]

The preceding descriptions of survivors are reassuring for struggling caregivers. You, too, can experience higher levels of confidence, self-worth, and spiritual strength from struggling through day-to-day crises to difficult caregiving settings. Ancient sayings, including one from China, claim opportunity lies in the midst of difficulty and crisis. **John**, one of the caregivers in our study, said, when asked about any positive results from his caregiving, "The inner strength that came from working through the crises, and the satisfaction of knowing that I was doing all that was possible to help, made me more understanding of friends in this situation."

Guidelines for Survivors

- Survivors have a way of turning misfortune into good fortune. Caregivers can use this principle to advantage by asking themselves how they might see this situation more positively. They might, for example, see that they are receiving valuable experience so that when their caregiving experience is over they could be employed as a professional care manager, practical nurse, aide in a child-care center, or director of an adult day-care center. Caregivers might perceive themselves as stronger persons—better able to endure frustration, disappointment, and bitterness. There is also the possibility of experiencing the pride of accomplishment for doing a difficult task, or the satisfaction of making a social contribution. Look back over your experience of caregiving, or your fantasies of future caregiving, and ask, *Were there instances when I perceived good things coming out of bad situations? What did I learn about myself that was useful? What new strengths did I acquire?*

- As a caregiver in difficult circumstances, you can learn more about your style of reacting to adversity. On one hand, do you respond typically, for example, with emotional outbursts, blaming others, or blaming yourself? Do you tend to react to adversity with detachment or feelings of being a victim of fate of conspiracy? On the other hand, is your response one of accepting the challenge and mobilizing your determination to see the positive possibilities? Have you ever responded with, "Why did this happen to a good person like me? If God loved me, why did he do this to me? Why am I always so unlucky?"
- Bite your lip as a symbol of your determination to be a survivor. Say to yourself, "I am a survivor! I can make a difference! I can change!" **Lois**, from our survey, said to the interviewer, "This experience has made me stronger. At first I didn't think I could last, but I said to myself, 'Hang in there, Lois; I know you can do it. You can really help this family survive this crisis.' "

Caregivers Who Function Optimally

Another approach to self-care it to look at the characteristics of people who have cared for themselves well and have achieved high levels of functioning. Charles Garfield studied characteristics of outstanding artists, government leaders, sports figures, and professionals.[6] Apart from the natural talent factor, you will note that these qualities can be acquired by most of us.

Qualities of Optimally Functioning Caregivers

- Strong internal motivation; self-starting, committed to exceed previous achievement.

- Take risks but do not act impulsively; move beyond the comfort zone.
- Visualize how an action can be performed and rehearse it mentally.
- Relax frequently and sleep on ideas to let them incubate.
- Build family and friendship support networks.
- Focus on those skills essential for excellence; do not try to be all things to all people.
- Manage time effectively; delegate; focus on essential tasks.
- Reflect and take time out often to think.
- Engage in physical activity.
- Generalize and synthesize rather than judge an idea or plan.
- Tolerate confusion, chaos, and ambiguity without stress.
- Welcome challenge.

Optimal performers work hard, but they work efficiently. They are not compulsive workaholics who often spend too much time on nonessential trivia. They work smoothly and take restful and creative break periods.

Becoming an Optimal Performer

Try on the preceding list for fit. Which qualities do you think you already have to a large degree? (Mark them with an X.) Which would you want to acquire? (Mark them with a check.) If you decline to do this inventory, so be it. Accept yourself as you are, and do the best you can each day, one day at a time. It would be a serious mistake to set high goals and then feel frustrated and inadequate because you could not achieve them.

Varieties of Care

Variety of Settings

Caregivers are a varied group of folks. It is difficult to describe a typical primary caregiver. We will experience an increasing need for primary caregivers because older adults are living longer. The over-eighty-five group is the fastest-growing, ratewise, of any group in the United States. This means that we can expect increasing numbers of frail and disabled elderly. At the same time, there are fewer children to serve as caregivers. Life expectancy is rising also, leaving more of us around to be cared for. According to the National Institute on Aging, life expectancy in the United States is expected to rise to 85.9 for men and 91.5 for women by 2040.[7]

The average caregiver is in the mid- to upper forties, employed, and often living with spouse and children. Sixty-six percent are married. The average age of a wife caring for her husband is sixty-five, and 30 percent are over the age of seventy-four.[8] The same national studies report wide variations in age, employment status, and time devoted to caregiving. Seventy-five percent of caregivers are women. One-fourth of the caregivers say they were caregivers because they had no choice—there was no one else.

Long-Term Care

Long-term care facilities and professional home caregiving agencies are increasing rapidly, but cost of such care makes it unrealistic for most families, even for the few with long-term care insurance. It is a myth, however, that most families abandon their elderly relatives to public assistance. Many middle-aged children give their parents care willingly, at first, but reluctantly later, when they experience the strain of the complex roles cited earlier in the chapter. As the elderly parent begins to require round-the-clock care, caregivers feel caught in a dilemma. They want to do their duty to their parents yet also want to escape the increasing demands of care.

The working middle-aged child sometimes leaves his or her job to care for the elderly parent or disabled child. New federal legislation, known as the Family Leave Law, will give caregivers more flexibility for work and care responsibilities. Most elderly parents do not want to live with their children, but health circumstances and finances often force them to do so.

Economics of Caregiving

Marginal incomes. Since most caregivers are women in their middle years, many of you are single parents. You want to be masters of your own lives and have sufficient money to live a comfortable life. The reality, however, is that single women caregivers often have little or no income unless they are employed or under Social Security. Few have pensions, and many care for persons who have only Social Security income.

The few who have incomes from employment can hire care managers or some supplemental home care and respite services, but the majority of women caregivers are unpaid full-time workers, many of whom live at or below the poverty level. In 1995 median income for women in the United States who are sixty-five or older was $8,500 a year, compared to older men's median of $15,000.[9] According to data compiled by the Older Women's League, 40 percent of older women living alone live at or near the poverty level.

The sudden money drain. **George and Judy** have just retired on comfortable pensions. Soon afterward, Judy's eighty-three-year-old mother went rapidly downhill physically. It was tacitly understood among the family that Judy, the newly retired daughter, would be the primary caregiver. Judy invited her mother into her home to save travel time and expense. George and Judy had not anticipated these extra expenses in their retirement planning. Her mother's Social Security income and Medicare did not come close to covering the extra costs of her care. Judy's unemployed brother helped some, but he was living close to the poverty level himself. Thus, George and Judy were catapulted from a comfortable retirement into marginal poverty.

The problems of pooling retirement incomes appear easy to manage compared to the economic drain of care outside the home. Even if full care is provided in the single caregiver's home, she risks poverty with increasing costs and loss of income through quitting her job. She also risks her own security by inability to contribute to her retirement fund.

Cost of renovation. Some of the added costs incurred when a care receiver moves into your home are the numerous alternations that must be made. Some of these changes are added railings, grab bars, ramps, nonskid rugs and furniture, and accessible shelves. Usually, plumbing changes such as special showers are also needed.

Financial anxieties. Financial concerns haunt both providers and receivers. Receivers often fear they are running out of funds, even though in reality they may be fairly well off. Conversely, the receiver's pride and independent spirit may mislead the caregiver into thinking that everything is all right when he or she is actually spending down to the last dollar.

Leonard's situation illustrates. He lived alone in an apartment. He had been independent for years, with only a younger sister to check on his condition occasionally. He kept his finances to himself all this time. His sister became suspicious when she noticed his empty refrigerator and almost bare cupboards. Her questions about money brought vehement denial and confusing answers. She brought food to him for a while and asked his neighbor to keep an eye on him. The neighbor called one day soon to report that her brother was acting strangely. Leonard's sister came over to confront her brother about giving up his apartment. Over his protests she finally got him to try a group home nearby. His sister took over as the primary caregiver for his business affairs. The first thing she did was obtain a durable power-of-attorney to manage his affairs.

Durable power of attorney. This is a legal document, usually added to the care recipient's will, to give you, the caregiver, the authority to make medical and other life-care decisions for your patient when he or she is unable to do so. For example, you may need authority to hospitalize and pay from your patient's funds, or you may need to sell property he or she no longer needs. Since you must have your care receiver's signature, this step needs to be taken while he or she is still able and willing to sign. The whole family should be in agreement to give you this power. This document will add much to your peace of mind.

Family financial planning conference. Frank talk together as a family about financial resources is essential for a smooth care situation. Laying the topic of finances on the table by all concerned will reduce sources of conflict later. Fears about running out of money can be aired. Concerns about provisions in the patient's will can be discussed. The delicate question of when it will become necessary for the caregiver to take over management of the receiver's finances can be covered in such a family conference. For example, who will manage the checking account, pay the bills, and file the tax returns?

Keeping records. Even though it would be an onerous task, keeping records of care expenditures, major financial decisions, and contract copies would save much grief at a later date. Such records would be helpful in applying for entitlements and services, as well as keeping family suspicions and rumors controlled.

Multicultural Caregiving Perspectives

With the large numbers of ethnic minority persons in industrialized countries, it is important to recognize differences in caregiving attitudes and responsibilities toward frail and disabled persons of all ages. We have been struck by the diversity of ethnic groups now living in urban environments. Attitudes about who is responsible for caring for older persons, children, and the disabled vary greatly, but the practice of caregiving has broad similarities. Our data are based on many years of studying multicultural issues, extended living in other cultures, and recent interviews with representatives of various groups on how they perceive the nature of caregiving in their groups.

At one time, most ethnic minority groups took care of older adults, disabled children, and their sick relatives of all ages in the nuclear family circle. In some societies, it was the extended family that looked after all the sick and abandoned children and adults in the village. The elders, especially, were treated with respect as wise and valued members of the family; they were not treated as burdens, which is a more common contemporary attitude. Even now, there are some family groups living in urban settings that not only take care of their own until death but also provide the bedridden with meaningful family tasks to give them a feeling of worth. Other elder family members still are regarded as the custodians of family history and cultural heritage.

Family Care Traditions

While many persons of African, Native American, Asian, or Hispanic descent have adopted the practices of the larger population, they still cling to the ideal of family care for the frail, sick, and disabled of all ages. Utilization of professional caregiving services is an indication that the caregiver was not assuming proper responsibility. It is also the federal policy of the United States to provide assistance to families so that the disabled member can stay at home as long as possible. This is not only sound fiscal policy, but it is also more humane than the trend toward "warehousing" the disabled in long-term care facilities. This feeling of responsibility for one's own family members also makes the final decision to place the disabled or dysfunctional family member in a long-term care setting painfully difficult.

Family Expectations of the Caregivers

What complicates caregiving for the ethnic minority member is the tradition of expecting the eldest or single daughter to be the primary care provider. **Anna**'s situation is an example. Being the middle-aged single daughter, she was expected to care for her aging parents. Anna was very angry that she was pressured into spending most of her middle adult life in caregiving, but her anger was increased when her three married older brothers and sisters got off free of caregiving duties. Anna's anger was furthered by the fact that she felt that her siblings did not pay their fair share of the costs.

Negative Stereotypes

An additional complication for minority caregivers is the legacy of racism and negative stereotypes that often leads them to feel inadequate or angry. If the caregiver is of a race different from that of the recipient of the care, for example, there may not be open prejudice but an invisible veil that reflects the racism of the surrounding society. Caregivers may be blind to its presence, but it is there.

Considering the condition discussed above, what is a caregiver to do?

1. First admit the possibility that you have ethnic or racial bias. Then try to become more aware of its presence.
2. Maintain close contact with the other person so you know each other on a personal basis. Then you can see each other as human beings with common goals and problems.
3. Strive for equal status in the relationship, since much prejudice comes from unequal power. This may mean one of the persons working on empowering the other as much as possible. An example is an effort to redress a master/servant sort of relationship.

Sally was a minority caregiver serving a handicapped older Caucasian couple. Especially the man treated Sally disrespectfully by making snide remarks about her racial background. While she addressed the couple as Mr. and Mrs. by their family names, they treated her in a patronizing manner and addressed her by her first name, never as Miss Sally. She finally confronted the couple about their patronizing and insulting manner. The couple, being dependent on Sally and fearful of losing her, brought her more into their activities, including meals together. They started treating her increasingly like a family member, and in the process became better acquainted. In getting to know one another, they developed more respect and appreciation for Sally a person, as well as a valued caregiver.

Generational Differences

While current generations do not carry out caregiving responsibilities as conscientiously as earlier, traditional families once did, their respect for elders and compassion for disabled persons is still present.[10] A strong reason for the differences in family support is socioeconomic. "Filial piety" has been a strong moral obligation upon younger members to care for and respect older members of the group. In many cultures, this support for older members was expected from the younger folks and was considered a kind of social insurance. In modern urban environments, families do not have the resources or extended family connections to carry out their traditional responsibilities. If you are caring for an elderly Hispanic patient, you might find the film *Barriers* useful in understanding his or her problems.

A Rosier Future in Sight

The research on caregiving emphasizes the complexity, variation, and heavy burden of caregiving. Even though the role is demanding, it offers satisfaction of important needs to be compassionate and helpful. Through this service, caregivers can experience greater meaning to their existence. They can look forward to the future of caregiving with greater confidence, knowing that the task will be easier. The keys to this rosier future are self-care and knowing how to access community services. With recent widespread media attention to the plight of the "forgotten caregiver," increasing attention of health-care agencies, and growing governmental programs, there is hope for a brighter future of recognition and support. Just the expansion of respite care alone has improved the lot of the caregiver immeasurably.

Special skills are needed to become a survivor and to function optimally. Chapter 2 presents a survival kit of coping skills.

Notes

1. Mary Morrissey (ed.), "More Grandparents Raising Grandchildren," *Counseling Today,* January 1997, p. 10.
2. Lawrence Brammer, "Evaluation of Project Access: AARP Region X and Gerontological Society of America" (a study of consultants to caregivers), 1988.
3. C. Gilbert Wrenn, *Intelligence, Feeling, Caring: Some Personal Perceptions* (Greensboro, NC: Eric/Cass, 1996).
4. Al Siebert, *The Survivor Personality* (New York: Periger, 1996).
5. Victor Frankl, *The Doctor and the Soul* (New York: Knopf, 1969).
6. Charles Garfield, "Why Do Some People Outperform Others?" *Wall Street Journal,* January 12, 1982, p. 2.
7. Dorothy Coons and Nancy Mace, *Quality of Life in Long-Term Care* (Binghamton, NY: Haworth, 1996).
8. Michael Johnson, *Labor of Love: A Guide for Caregivers* (Seattle: AARP Project Access, 1988), p. 8b.
9. Family Survival Project—San Francisco, "Overworked, Underestimated" (research summary), Family Survival Project, 425 Bust St., Suite 500, San Francisco, CA 94108, p. 3. (They also publish a newsletter, *Update.*)
10. Shirley Lockery, "Caregiving among Racial and Ethnic Minority Elders," *Generations,* Fall/Winter, pp. 58–62.

Recommended Reading

AARP. *Miles Away and Still Caring.* Washington, DC: American Association of Retired Persons, 1994. (A guide for long-distance caregivers.)

Berman, Claire. *Caring for Yourself While Caring for Your Aging Parents.* New York: Henry Holt, 1996.

Carter, Rosalynn. *Helping Yourself Help Others.* New York: Times, 1994. (A report of the caregiver research and services of the Carter Institute in Atlanta.)

Coons, Dorothy, and Nancy Mace. *Quality of Life in Long-Term Care.* Binghamton, NY: Haworth, 1996.

Heath, Angela. *Care Log: A Planning and Organizing Aid for Long-Distance Caregivers.* San Luis Obispo, CA: Impact, 1994. (Balancing personal life and caregiving tasks.)

———. *Long-Distance Caregiving: A Survival Guide for Far-Away Caregivers.* San Luis Obispo, CA: Impact, 1995.

Horel, Zen, McKinney, Edward, and Williams, Michael. *Black Understanding Diversity and Service Needs.* Newberry Park, CA: Sage, 1990.

Lustbader, Wendy. *A Prescription for Caregivers: Take Care of Yourself.* A videotape of a lecture and a live audience of caregivers. Available for $92.31, including shipping, from Wendy Lustbader, 1917 25th Avenue East, Seattle, WA 98112.

Norris, Jane, ed. *Daughters of the Elderly.* Bloomington: Indiana University Press, 1988.

Roberts, Jeanne. *Taking Care of Caregivers.* Palo Alto, CA: Bull, 1991. (Written for dementia caregivers.)

Smith, Kerri. *Caring for Your Aging Parents.* San Luis Obispo, CA: Impact, 1994.

2
Survival of the Fittest

The caregiver is a person in most need of care.
—Maya Angelou, April 1997 speech

Caregivers as Skilled Copers

Are you a hardy coper? You probably are a fairly good coper now, or you would not have survived this far into adulthood. If you are new to caregiving or picture yourself as a future caregiver, you have time to sharpen those coping skills essential to survival. In this chapter we will give you a survival kit of skills—receiving support, managing stress, and changing negative thinking.

We present **Angela** as an example of a survivor. For ten years she has been caring for her husband, who suffers from progressive Parkinson's disease and cerebral artery problems, which have taken their toll. Yet she has coped well with the strain and her anticipatory grief. Angela went to work part-time so she could hire a part-time housekeeper and occasional home health worker and has joined a local church and finds that the program satisfies her spiritual needs. In addition, Angela turned their spare bedroom into a hideaway for herself. She continues with her bimonthly support group meetings. Her parting statement was, "I'm trying to cope with a difficult, deteriorating condition, but I think I have the strength and skill now to make the best of a bad situation."

Coping is an active approach to managing change. What kinds of change? We mean ordinary events such as suffering an illness, having an accident, becoming a crime victim, getting fired, and losing a relationship. Even positive changes that are chosen (vacations, retirement, marriage, promotions, and achievement) can be extremely stressful. So, change can move you forward or it can hold you back.

Useful Coping Attitudes

Suzann Kobassa's research on coping identified the qualities of what she called "hardy copers." These survivor qualities were the 3Cs—control, challenge, and commitment.[1]

- *Control.* Control is the belief that you are in charge of your life and this problem situation. You **act** as if you are in control. Self-control, then, becomes an important survival trait, and you would no longer have the need to see yourself as a helpless victim. There are situations that you cannot always control, such as unavoidable accidents. Skillful copers, however, believe that they are mainly responsible for what happens to them. Fate and divine intervention take a backseat. **Blake**'s attitude is illustrative here: "I grew up thinking that my life was controlled by destiny. Now I realize that I am the one who is calling the signals; I am not a helpless pawn on life's fateful chessboard." In your moments of respite from care, we suggest that you reflect on the question: To what extent are you, divine power, and impersonal chance controlling your life?
- *Challenge.* Looking at a difficult problem as a challenge—an interesting problem to solve—is the second quality of a skillful coper. Effective copers

welcome change in their lives as a push to growth and as an escape from a comfortably boring rut. **Nora,** one of our interviewees, said, "Some days I don't know if I will make it. There is so much to do; but I'm taking these challenges one day at a time."
- *Commitment.* If you are a good coper, you are committed. You are focused on the tasks of caregiving and stay the course. You believe that what you are doing is important, and you have clear goals for your life. **Opel's** outlook illustrates commitment: "Taking care of Mother is my life. She gave me my life, and now the least I can do is make her life as rich as possible. Right now I believe that caring for her is the most important thing I can do."

Attitudes toward Change

- *Change is normal.* Viewing change as a normal part of living helps you cope with the strain of those changes. Perhaps you have noted that as you think about the changes in your life, your distress increases. This is so especially when you view change as a difficult problem to solve, a curse, an unlucky event, or even a conspiracy. Realistically, not all life changes can be viewed as challenges or be welcomed as opportunities. They can be viewed as undesirable, but normal, intrusions that must be taken in stride. In one of our survey interviews, **Albert** said, "When I suddenly was faced with long-term care for my mother, my first reaction was that God was punishing me. Then, after the cold sweat on my face dried, I realized that frailty in aging is a normal event that comes to all of us."
- *Change creates opportunities.* Caregiving produces many changes in your life. You can look beyond the

problems, crises, and challenges to see the opportunities that such changes present. Change often forces a novel way of responding, a new view of life, or a fresh way to look at this problem. Thus, disruption caused by change is an opportunity for creativity. The first requirement for such creativity to take place is shaking up your old way of thinking and acting. The resulting chaotic state is uncomfortable for you, so you resist change like a virus. You can also choose to shake up your life in small, tolerable amounts. This is the function of vacations, hobbies, and education. Change lifts you out of your everyday routines that tend to be boring or deadening. The unstable condition that follows opens you to new possibilities for growth. It is like soaking beans before you cook them. They must be softened first.

Potential Danger—Fight or Flight?

Assessing danger is a basic survival skill we share with all animals. Two researchers on coping, Richard Lazarus and Susan Folkman, found that when people are threatened by change or face a crisis they first assess the extent of danger. This assessing skill is used to determine if the threat is indeed dangerous and then take action such as fight-or-flight. If the threat is not dangerous, just annoying, you may choose to avoid or ignore it. If you judge the threat to be a challenge, then you may choose to use your coping skill.[2]

We realize that this discussion sounds quite theoretical, so we will illustrate with the following example: **Donald**, a caregiver for five years, was told by his physician that he had advanced throat cancer. He immediately saw that this was not only a life-threatening diagnosis he could no longer ignore but also a threat to his caregiver role.

Being a skilled coper, he took the crisis as a challenge to apply what he knew about cancer, wellness, and alternative medicine. To him, it was a problem-solving challenge to do everything he could do prolong his life and to live as fully as he could during the remaining months or years.

Building and Using Support

Support consists of an attentive and caring presence and the communication of compassionate and understanding attitudes. Support means that when you are in a state of crisis you can lean on the stronger, supportive person until you feel courageous and strong enough to provide your own internal support.

Values of Support

Giving emotional support to others helps your own peace of mind, care effectiveness, and life satisfaction. Receiving support is essential to your good mental and physical health. Support is help you receive from relatives, friends, and colleagues. It is informal, intermittent, and usually unsolicited. When support is organized into a system it becomes a network. Professional writings on helping relationships emphasize strongly that networks are very important means to help people in the process of change or planning change. An example is the task of making a decision to have your patient moved to a long-term care facility or from the facility back home. To use a network you would call people you know who have the experience in placing a relative in a care facility. You also would consult with physicians and gerontologists who are on your network. Then you would act, based upon your best judgment and tempered by the consensus of the experts.

Types of Support

- *Encouragement.* Emotional support takes the form of simple encouragement and strengthening of your determination to go on. The poet John Greenleaf Whittier expressed it well: "If there be some weaker one, give me strength to help him on." In caregiving it is easy for you to become discouraged, so receiving an encouraging word occasionally from family, health specialists, or the care receiver is welcome support. The care receivers get more hope, confidence, and courage for themselves in the exchange. This "round robin" of support, which makes both of you feel good, is facilitated by remarks that affirm, such as, "You are a wonderful trooper," or, "You are doing just great." Comments such as these are likely to trigger comparable responses from the patient who is competent to do so: "You are a good caregiver, too," or, "I really appreciate your good care." Giving examples of courage by well-known persons is encouraging also. Telling your wheelchair patient the story of past president Franklin D. Roosevelt's high achievements, even though he spent much of his adult life confined to a wheelchair, could be affirming.
- *A supportive presence.* Fear of saying the wrong thing discourages some caregivers from offering emotional support. You must realize that it is not so much what you say as it is your presence and attitude that are supporting. Just sitting with the person quietly is supportive.
- *Receiving compliments.* If your care receiver is offering encouragement to you, it is important to receive that supportive comment graciously. We emphasize this obvious point because some caregivers feel so undeserving and self-critical that they cannot accept a compliment. Do you respond to compliments with

self-deprecation and denial? If so, being aware of this tendency is the first step to change. This is a response that can be changed by smiling and saying, "Thank you," until a more natural acceptance of the compliment becomes comfortable.

- *Supportive touching and hugging.* How do you feel when a patient puts his or her hand on your shoulder or gives you a hug when you are hurting? Most of the time it feels very good, but there are those times when you do not want anyone close to you, much less one who wants to hug. How do you know what your care receiver wants? Look at her or his misty eyes or downcast face, and then take a chance. When in doubt about what people want in the way of supportive touching, ask them! If you do not know the person well or you are uncertain of his or her response, a light hand on your shoulder or your grasping a hand and moving in closer conveys the patient's acceptance or rejection of your support efforts. In any case, it is prudent and ethical to respect people's boundaries. An important guideline, however, is to know your own motives well. It is important also to know that your sincere intentions to convey support may be misinterpreted. For example, there are different intentions conveyed by touch—greeting, friendship, healing, intimacy, power, and sexuality. The first three are reasonably safe supportive motives, but you must be careful not to unconsciously convey power or seductive intent with your affectionate acts, under the guise of support.

A Multicultural View of Support

The issue of touching is a good example of the need for multicultural knowledge. In some contexts, touching the other person would be offensive, just as in some cultures they would be offended if you did not use touch to convey greetings, social acceptance, or support. Whether or not a supportive act is acceptable depends on cultural expectations, whether you are a member of that ethnic group, and whether you are in a public or private setting. The main guidance here is to be informed about how various cultures deal with issues of intimacy, privacy, and support.

Similar statements can be made about kissing. In some cultures, as in the Middle East, men kiss each other in public as a greeting, but touching between men and women is done only in the privacy of the home. In U.S. and most European groups, men are much less demonstrative than women. As caregivers, we need to understand these differences in our care receivers so we do not satisfy our needs for affection at the risk of their discomfort.

Support for Caregivers, Too

Caregivers need supportive touch and hugs from their care receivers, too. **Joyce**, a spousal caregiver, said, "Ever since my husband's illness began, I hug him and he ever so slightly pushes me away. I really miss being held." Compassionate touch can be healing and restore energy and alertness to both giver and receiver. A healing touch releases the inner wisdom of the body. Health-care workers use it frequently, so you might wish to try it in your caregiving ministrations. Touching for healing purposes has become a common nursing practice.

Seek support to regain control when you think you are falling apart. Find a friend or a member of your support group to talk it over with you. If these self-help steps are not sufficient, we suggest you call a professional counselor for support.

Guidelines for Building and Sustaining Support

- Make changes in your network much as you do when revising your holidays greeting card list. For example, should someone be added or dropped? Do some people take support from you but give little in return? Should you add people to provide a special kind of support, such as someone you could laugh or cry with or someone you could call at three o'clock in the morning?
- How do you handle encouragement and appreciation with your family and your care recipient? Do you tell them you remember and appreciate them? Do you encourage yourself and give yourself a frequent pat on the back? Just the knowledge that you have made a difference in someone's life is a kind of self-appreciation. Reflect on it! Celebrate it! Charles Dickens noted that "no one is useless in this world who lightens the burden of it for anyone else."
- If you are new at caregiving, find a mentor. This is an experienced person who might be willing to advise you, comfort you, and be your advocate to access social services. This should be a person you trust and with whom you feel comfortable.

Coping with Hassles and Stressors

Caregiver Stressors

By this time you probably are an expert in recognizing and describing your caregiving stressors. Therefore, we will concentrate on what you can do to manage not only the big stressful events but also the little hassles that soon wear you down. For example, the CareNet Study indicated that providing personal hygiene for care receivers was the most stressful task for caregivers. It was physically demanding and emotionally traumatic.[3]

New caregivers face several immediate risks: demands and criticisms from family members, isolation from friends, perceived loss of control of their lives, and economic strain due to loss of employment are just a few. In the worst-case scenario, the new caregivers may be baffled by troublesome patients' behavior, such as screaming, violence, wandering, and dependence on the caregiver for daily living assistance. Chronic depression and suspicion are not easy to face either. These situations contribute to the feeling of being overwhelmed or, at least, stressed out.

There is *good stress*, the kind you choose that is stimulating and sometimes pleasant. Performing before an audience and climbing mountains are stressful, but they provide joy of achievement. They add excitement, novelty and challenge to what could otherwise be a dull existence. What tasks in your caregiving routine could be considered good stress?

The kind of stress we will discuss is unplanned and sometimes overwhelming and painful. You will recognize the signs easily—pounding heart, sweaty hands, rapid and shallow breathing. Not visible is the hormone rush in our blood, narrowing vessels, increased blood pressure, and increased mental alertness. In ancient times these responses were essential to survival, but now they are largely dysfunctional, because they keep one in a mental and physical state of uproar. You still need some signals, however, to warn of threatening or embarrassing situations; over time, however, a persistent state of alertness due to stress is bad for your health.

Now, think of your caregiving situation. Is it like any of the following scenarios?

Christa became a primary caregiver to her elderly mother in Christa's home. This was not a sudden change of role for Christa, since she was also a caregiver for two children and a working husband. Her mother suffered moderate dementia and *transition shock* from the move to Christa's home. Mother was irritable and demanding, blaming Christa for taking her out of her own home. Christa felt caught among the additional demands of two school-age children, a husband (who helped with some chores), full-time employment as a teacher's aide, and now care of her mother, too. The family of four take turns being at home with Mother, but the main burden falls on Christa. They are barely making it financially, with two modest incomes and high expenses. After two weeks, Christa began to feel the pressure and said she was not sure how long she could take it. She began to experience headaches and fatigue due to loss of sleep. If you were Christa's mentor, what would you advise?

Joanna moved to town two weeks ago. She brought along her elderly father, who had been in long-term care in their former city. She wanted him near her, and to reduce the costs of his care she took him into her home. She thought she would care for him full-time and not seek employment again for a while. While the caregiving went smoothly those first weeks, the overall hassles began to take their toll. Finding a new physician, a real estate lawyer to help with the property transfer, and locating shopping, car repair, and cleaning shops were major chores. Her car was balky, her teeth needed attention, and she misplaced her car keys on the day she had two appointments.

The stresses of the move for herself and her father were taken in stride. However, in combination with the tasks of getting settled and the little things that went wrong those first two weeks, she was severely stressed. She began to have trouble sleeping and eating, was irritable and short-tempered with her father, and began losing things—papers, keys, clothes, and appointments. The hassles were accumulating faster than she could deal with them. If you were her mentor, what would you say she should do?

Lyle has been taking care of his aging father who, until recently, was fairly self-sufficient. The two of them got along well and Lyle got much satisfaction out of his role as caregiver. He was worried about whether he should keep his job if his father needed more intensive care. Lyle experienced considerable stress in his work because he and his supervisor could not get along. They were in constant conflict over deadlines. Lyle came home almost every night tense and tired. What advice would you give to Lyle, who likes and does well in his caregiving role but is stressed because of his job pressures?

Strategies for Stress Management

Successful stress management requires three lines of attack. The first is changing the caregiving life situation, as in Christa's predicament with competing forces of care, family, and work. Christa might arrange for more family help or cut her commitments, for example. The second approach is to change the overwhelming forces and hassles outside of caregiving responsibility, as in Joanna's life. The third approach, illustrated by Lyle, is to change one's self. Lyle's stress seemed to come mainly from conflicts on his job. He might decide to be more careful about honoring deadlines and to work on better communication with his supervisor.

Part of the third strategy of changing yourself is to develop stronger coping skills to tolerate higher levels of stress over time without burning out. This is good prevention strategy and what stress expert Donald Meichenbaum called *stress inoculation*.[4] The following guidelines and suggestions will help you to achieve this goal.

Surviving Holidays

Holidays are an especially stressful time for families. One stress expert, Allen Elkin estimates that 43 percent of persons get depressed, anxious, or severely upset over the major holidays.[5] Your caregiving duties during holidays are most likely affected by two streams of stress. One is the response to the usual holiday hassles—shopping, preparing food, wrapping presents, and entertaining friends and relatives. The frenetic pace that pervades homes accounts for at least half of the stress. The second major source of stress is from memories and unfinished emotional business of the family. There are sad memories for some, such as memories of a missing family member and the recall of happy events of the past. Anniversaries are especially difficult. Another source is unrealistic expectations, as in anticipating an unlikely gift or expecting the holiday to be full of frivolity and good cheer. It is often not a happy time.

Guidelines for Managing Holiday Stress

- See the absurdity in the frantic activities and laugh about them.
- Rehearse what you regard as realistic expectations.
- Support relatives who have painful memories.
- Avoid overplanning; keep plans simple; buy and wrap your gifts early.
- Bury old emotional hatchets before the events.
- Keep groups and parties small.

Guidelines for Managing Stress in General

This is a supplement to the list in the previous chapter for preventing burnout.

- Identify how you respond to stressful situations. How do you respond typically to interruptions, harassment, hassles, incomplete tasks, deadlines, and criticism? What does your body tell you? What are your body's points of vulnerability to sustained stress (stomach, heart, lungs, muscles, head)?
- Learn a relaxation technique or strengthen a favorite method you use now, such as focusing on your breathing. Learning to relax the large muscle groups through a progressive relaxation method is easy to do and is effective in reducing tension.[6] You carry your stressful memories in your tense muscles, so relaxation exercises are your answer. Your goal is to achieve the relaxation response whenever you say to yourself, "Relax!" Get a tape on facilitating relaxation, which you can keep next to your bed. Play it to go to sleep quickly after an exhausting and tension-filled day. The voices on these tapes are soothing and quieting. They are filled with suggestions and images, such as colorful sunsets and warm beaches.
- Imagery makes use of your imagination to reduce tension. In addition to visualizing your body in a relaxed state, you can think of yourself as a limp dishcloth or bowl of gelatin. You can take a mental trip to a place of joy, peace, contentment, and play. You can go to your favorite beach, for example, to feel the warm sun on your skin and the soft breezes caressing your body.
- Practice stopping your thoughts instantly. You simply say to yourself, "Stop," and after some practice you will be able to stop your line of thought and focus on putting your body into a relaxed state. Tense muscles reflect tense thoughts and worries, so get rid of the troublesome thoughts.

- Laugh heartily and you will not feel the pain of stress. Follow the guidelines of the section on humor that appears later in this book. Forcing out a pinched smile is a start, but you really need a belly laugh to do the job right.
- Note the time traps that you may have fallen into—letting others set your priorities and control your time and viewing yourself as a victim or door mat. Recall the discussion on controlling your life. Regain that control over your time and your life. You may need to do some soul-searching to affirm whether your personal style of time management resembles the turtle, the rabbit, or the race horse. It is important to remember that time management is based on self-management.
- Examine the messages you are giving yourself about time pressures. Change them before it is too late. Examples are: "I must finish my work before I can read my book or play the piano"; "I must always respond to requests for help"; "Time is precious, so I must use every minute carefully"; and "It is selfish of me to put myself first." Experienced caregivers call these examples part of the *Messiah trap*—the tendency to play God, trying to meet everyone's needs with perfection and selflessness.
- Take *down time* for solitude and contemplation and meditation. These actions are necessary to get in touch with your deeper feelings and gain perspective on your life.
- Consider things that could be done in advance to prevent a crisis. Exchanging telephone numbers with friends and neighbors, having your emergency and social service numbers handy, checking wills, trusts, and bank accounts, and securing extra car and house keys, for example.

Changing Negative Thoughts

Identifying Your Negative Thoughts

You conduct fantasy conversations with yourself naturally every day, especially if you have few people to talk with. Thus, you have the foundation for the coping skill of changing your negative, self-defeating, and dysfunctional conversations into constructive thoughts. You must believe that you can change your actions, starting with your thoughts and feelings. You must also believe that you have enormous power over your thoughts and your behavior. Now, you are ready to look at the coping skill of changing negative thoughts.

Becoming Aware of Negative Thoughts

Step 1. The first step is to be aware that you have negative thoughts that are defeating your best caring efforts and stunting your own psychological growth.

Step 2. Then it is easy to identify the specific self-defeating message you are giving yourself. For example, you might say to yourself on one of those bad days. *I can't do this task anymore; it's killing me. I'm really not cut out to be a caregiver.* While it may be true that you are not the world's premier caregiver, nevertheless, you probably are not as bad as you think you are. Since you probably do not make self-statements like this aloud, it is subvocal and hidden from you. So, ask yourself, *What am I saying to myself that is making me so upset about caregiving?* Another example, when you are anxious about going to your support group, might be: *What am I telling myself about this meeting that is making me so anxious?* Another example might be, when you forgot to give your patient his or her medication on time, *What is this act of forgetting telling me about my feelings toward my care receiver?* Sometimes forgetting is due to perceiving the task as unpleasant or disliking the person.

Evaluating Your Self-Talk

When you are clearly aware of what messages are going on in your head, you can examine the self-talk for distortions. These twisted self-messages are rooted in your need to feel miserable, sad, or punitive toward yourself or others, for example. Now you must be willing to examine these thoughts forthrightly and be open to changing them. Examples of such extreme thoughts in the depressed person are: *I am a no-good person; I can't do anything. It's hopeless.* In this evaluation step, you may ask several questions:

1. Did I draw a conclusion for which there is little or no evidence? For example, if you say you cannot do anything, you are overlooking the evidence that you can do some things and do them very well.
2. Did I magnify the feeling, problem, or thought? Thinking you are a no-good person respresents an extreme judgment. You may have some undesirable qualities, but thinking you are a bad person distorts the reality that you have redeeming qualities.
3. Did I oversimplify the situation? Rigid thinking in absolutes—such as good/bad, success/failure, and right/wrong—without considering all the in-between positions tends to oversimplify the situation. If you say, "I'm a failure as a caregiver," it probably means you have rigid standards and acknowledge only two categories—success and failure. It is easy to use labels such as *failure* in a negative self-evaluation.

4. Have I overgeneralized by using only one or two examples of my conclusions? You might say that your day was "a real bust" and that nothing came out well. Did you base this statement selectively on two instances when things did not go right: the dog tracked mud all over the carpet and your cat vomitted twice. These are not pleasant events to deal with, but they are very limited bases for concluding that the day was a bust. Watch out for words such as *never, always, can't,* and *should*.

Additional Examples of Common Self-Defeating Talk

Every culture has a list of illogical, biased, and irrational beliefs that result in emotional distress. Caregivers are as vulnerable as anyone, so we suggest that you use the following list (adapted from Albert Ellis and M. E. Bernard[7]) as a guide to search your thoughts. Some of these unspoken beliefs that are common in Western European traditions are:

- It is necessary that we be loved and approved by everyone.
- Certain acts are wrong, wicked, or villainous, and those who perform them should be punished.
- It is just terrible, even catastrophic, when things do not go the way we would like them to go.
- Our unhappiness is caused by external events.
- We need someone stronger than ourselves upon whom to rely.
- We need to be competent, adequate, and skilled in all possible domains.
- Once something strongly affects our life, it should affect us indefinitely.

- It is important to change other people in the direction we would like them to go.
- We have little control over our emotions.
- If we do not do it, it will not get done.
- We must help everyone who needs us.
- If we refuse this request, he or she will think we are terrible people.
- We must try harder.

To which of these beliefs do you subscribe? Look at the absurd or irrational beliefs in these statements. How would you change them? Do you have some irrational beliefs that are not on the list?

Restructuring Your Self-Talk

Now that you can pick out the irrational flaws in your self-descriptive statements, we will look at ways to change those beliefs. The skill involved is in examining the negative statement and asking, *How can I change this into a more realistic and affirming description?* It is tempting to flip all the way over from a self-critical to an extremely optimistic and uplifting trait. For example: *I am an extremely likable person.* Modest gains are the rule. Since it has taken a lifetime to acquire the negative thinking habits, they are not likely to change in one attempt.

In the earlier example of the caregiver's self-depreciation, you need to ask how you can replace this negative self-evaluation with one that is more positive. To make this change, you write a positive statement and then repeat it to yourself. You might say, "I knew that caregiving would be a tough assignment, and there are parts of it that I don't like; nevertheless, it is an opportunity to do good work and serve the community." Another example is, "When I finish my caregiver practical-nurse training at Toulouse Community College, I will be able to find a better job," instead of, "I'm so old now that I don't think I'll ever be able to find a decent job."

This method of restructuring your thinking is not easy. It takes much practice. The ultimate goal for doing this thinking change is to change your behavior. If you think confident self-affirming thoughts, you will act confidently. It is that simple.

Guidelines for Changing Thoughts

Practice *cognitive ecology* regularly.[8] For example, set aside ten minutes each week to recall all the self-defeating and negative self-descriptive statements you made during the week. Root them out ruthlessly! Scrutinize them carefully and apply the criteria listed earlier for evaluating self-talk. For example, were there times when other people did not behave the way you wanted them to and you got upset? Did you try to change them? Did you think that you had to be happy all week? Did you think other people made you unhappy? Did you use the word *should* often? Did you discount your personal strengths and dwell on the weaknesses? Did you make dire predictions about the future?

Rewrite these negative statements into a more affirming, positive style, replacing unreasonable self-talk. Be kind to yourself. Forgive yourself. Praise yourself for trying this difficult task.

Avoid asking "why questions" as in, *Why do I think this way?* This leads to frustrating dead-end ruminations. Ask instead, *What am I saying to myself that is upsetting me, and how can I change my thinking?*

Welcome to the Hardiness Hall of Fame

We defined *skilled copers* as being in control of their lives, viewing problems as challenges, and being fully committed to caregiving as a way of life. Good caregivers are masters of personal change. They welcome change as an opportunity for personal growth. Skillful copers can cushion themselves to psychological dangers by building personal support networks, facing annoying hassles, and mastering grueling stress.

If you apply the thirteen caregiver self-help survival skills and attitudes successfully, in the course of studying this book, you qualify for the Hardy Caregiver Hall of Fame. You will realize the rewards of greater love, wellness, and energy. You will experience also the deep satisfaction of a caregiving job well done. Best wishes to you on the beginning of your journey.

While this chapter focused on self-help skills for coping, the next chapter emphasizes tapping your inner resources of humor and spirituality.

Notes

1. Suzann Kobassa, "Stressful Life Events, Personality, and Health," *Journal of Personality and Social Psychology* 37 (1979): 1–11.
2. Richard Lazarus and Susan Folkman, *Stress, and Appraisal, and Coping* (New York: Springer, 1984).
3. Rosalynn Carter, *Helping Yourself Help Others* (New York: Times, 1994). (The Carter Institute sponsored and conducted the CareNet study "Caregivers and Caregiving in West Central Georgia," 1996).
4. Donald Meichenbaum, *Stress Inoculation Training* (Elmsford, NY: Pergamon, 1985).

5. Allen Elkin, *"Holiday Stress,"* Fox TV broadcast, December 5, 1996.
6. Lawrence Brammer, *How to Cope with Life Transitions: The Challenge of Personal Change* (New York: Hemisphere, 1991). (See chapter on relaxation methods.)
7. Albert Ellis and M. E. Bernard (eds.), *Clinical Application of Rational-Emotive Therapy* (New York: Plenum, 1985).
8. Donald Meichenbaum, *Cognitive Behavior Modification* (New York: Plenum, 1977).

Recommended Reading

Brammer, Lawrence. *Coping with Life Transitions.* New York: Hemisphere, 1991.

Monat, Alan, and Richard Lazarus. *Stress and Coping: An Anthology,* 3rd ed. New York: Columbia University Press, 1991.

New York Alzheimer Resource Center. *Caring: A Family Guide.* New York: New York Alzheimer Resource Center, 1994.

O'Connor, Kathleen, and Joyce Brothers. *The Alzheimer's Caregiver: Strategies for Support.* Seattle: University of Washington Press, 1995.

PART II
Knowing Your Inner Resources

3
Knowing Your Inner Strengths

Give me a sense of humor, Lord.
Give me the grace to see a joke,
To get some pleasure out of life
And pass it on to other folks.
— Alex MacLeod, editor, *Seattle Times*

Caregivers need inner strengths to survive. These inner strengths include mainly a deep spirituality and a lively sense of humor. Each springs from the deep well of your being and, when tapped, gives your caregiving more energy, purpose, and direction. Spiritual awareness and humor also lead to a greater sense of well-being.

Spiritual Resources

What Is Spirituality?

Everyone is spiritual, in the sense that spirit literally means "life" or "breath." It concerns the big life questions that we all face. Each of us has a different view of spirituality, however. This is the reason it is so difficult to define. We offer our ideas here as a challenge, to clarify and expand your views of the spiritual life.

Joseph Campbell, the eminent anthropologist, claimed that the challenge of spirituality is to live life to its fullest.[1] We will describe some elements of spirituality that clarify the big questions of life and what it means to live life to its fullest. For example, spirituality raises such questions as: "Why are you here?"; "What makes life meaningful and worthwhile?"; "What gives you purpose and hope?"; "What is the meaning of suffering?"; "Where do good and evil come from?"; "How do people relate to each other in the community?"; "What is vitally important to you?"; and "What beliefs and myths sustain you?" Finally, the big identity question is, "Who are you?"

Elements of Spirituality

Answers to the preceding questions define your spirituality and offer some "boxes" to put your "spirits" in. The answers represent your personal version of meaning and purpose, morality and ethics, intentional community, basic beliefs, core values, and identity. Then there is that special something that defines your unique sense of being. This aspect of your spiritual self defies description because words fail. It is a vague mysterious feeling—an awareness of a special center—a locus of soul. The fortunate ones get fleeting glimpses of this mystery at special times. These bits of awareness come at unpredictable moments, such as while watching a sunset, making love, offering a prayer, having a moving religious experience, giving birth, listening to a symphony, playing a sport, or cuddling a child.

If the spiritual experience described above is felt intensely, it could be, in Abraham Maslow's terms, a peak experience.[2] These experiences are occasional rapturous events accompanied by feelings of joy, unity, peace, mystery, and fulfillment. Examples of such unusual events are creating a piece of art, having a transformational religious experience, playing a stimulating game, and communing with unusual natural beauty in a sunset, mountain, or ocean waves. Thus, peak experiences are an important part of your spiritual life. Energy flows from these experiences, and they generate a sense of awe, belonging, intense self-awareness, and closeness with God. Even a busy caregiver can extract time to look at a shining star, shimmering moonlight on the water, fall leaves, or young children happily playing to get at least a taste of a peak experience.

Meaning in Spirituality

This aspect of spirituality is an especially important resource for caregivers. The question of why you are giving this care at this time of your life is bound to arise occasionally. This concern seldom is expressed to others, probably for fear of criticism about your questionable motivation. The majority of caregivers answer this question by saying to themselves, *It's there to do and I am the responsible person to do it, so no big deal.* Answers to this "why" question help to make sense of, and give purpose to, a caregiver's present life. This answer that "it's there to do" makes service a key to the meaning of life. "It was important to me to take care of Dad willingly—no regrets, no guilt," said **William**, one of our caregivers.

If this discussion of meaning as a part of spirituality is confusing or if the answers to your basic question of motivation are not clear, it would be prudent to discuss this issue with a trusted friend or counselor. It would not be mentally healthy, for example, to continue thinking that your caregiving tasks were involuntarily imposed on you and perceive your tasks as meaningless, punitive, onerous, or unimportant.

You probably see the same mental trap here that we see. There is a temptation to deal with meaning-of-life questions in a purely abstract, descriptive way. By contrast, the important question is: "What is the everyday experience of living that gives meaning?" It helps to see meaning in eating, working, cooking, cleaning, and body care, for example.

The meaningfulness of life must be discovered, of course, from your life experiences. You do not find meaning in a book, guru, therapist, or spiritual adviser—as attractive as these external sources might appear. This warning is not intended to exclude external resources that stimulate or facilitate your search for meaning and purpose, whether from religious institutions or unusually insightful and charismatic individuals.

Guidelines for Meaning

- *Learn the spiritual discipline of meditation.* Its purpose in the Buddhist tradition, for example, is to achieve physical relaxation, peace of mind, and temporary release from worldly cares and thinking processes. The goal is to achieve the state called *satori*, when the meaning of life emerges without effort. The meditating process is simple and nonmystical and is focused on natural breathing.

    1. Select a quiet place.
    2. Choose a comfortable sitting position.
    3. Focus on your breathing, being aware of your breath moving slowly in and out.
    4. Vocalize softly a nonsense syllable to help stay focused and keep out unwanted thoughts.
    5. Practice this process at least once a day for ten to fifteen minutes.

    In a short time you will see that this meditative process is helpful to relax and gain temporary respite from your cares. Prayer for some people is a form of meditation. When meditation is used as a spiritual practice, as in the Zen Buddhist, Christian, and Hebrew traditions, it facilitates giving up striving, peels off layers of cultural crust, and reduces worldly desires. Once you are in this meditative state, it is easier to incorporate a more structured practice, such as contemplation or prayer. In addition, taking a few moments a day to do the deep natural breathing is an effective centering method for instant relief from tension.

- *Practice the spiritual discipline of contemplation.* This involves a state of intense focus on a religious symbol or object, such as an altar, a cross, a star of David, a flower, special beads, a statue of Buddha or Christ, or a cathedral rose window. Then a flow of ideas, visions, or images emerges. The practice of contemplation has ancient roots and is a key part of all religious traditions. In a state of contemplation, the focus may be on the presence of God, Scripture passages, and spiritual rituals. While one result is the spiritual experience itself, it is expected also that the meanings that emerge can serve as guides to everyday life. An example is how the awareness of God dwelling in all people and all nature affects all life choices.

- *Study the spiritual practices of ethnic groups* that do not come from the mainstream of Judeo-Christian, Islamic, Buddhist, or Hindu traditions. Examples are Native Americans, diverse groups on the Indian subcontinent, and ancient Zoroastrian, Bahai, and Celtic groups. These traditions can make contributions that could enrich your spiritual ideas and practices.

Morals and Ethics

Morals. This aspect of spirituality is of keen interest to caregivers because your morals and ethics guide your everyday decisions on care. Your morals are those rules of personal behavior you have inherited from your family upbringing and community customs. Some, like the Ten Commandments and injunctions of the Koran, were institutionally codified and systematically taught. Obvious examples of guiding moral principles are honesty, integrity, justice, sobriety, and chastity. Caregivers are making judgments constantly about what is fair and what their obligations are to their care receivers.

When your recipient makes unfair demands, is vindictive, or makes false accusations, how to you react? It is tempting to be punitive or abusive, but our moral convictions and our love restrain us. Our morality also deters us from taking unfair advantage of a dependent person financially, emotionally, or physically.

Ethics. Ethics are refined social morals put in the form of precise behavioral guidelines. Examples for caregivers are: It is unethical to reveal confidential conversations to others or to sexually harass or abuse the person in our care. Ethical guidelines also remind us not only what *not to do*, but also what *to do*. For example, giving the best care possible is the great ethical imperative for caregivers. Involving care recipients in decisions affecting them is another example of ethical action. Encouraging a person to be as independent and empowered as possible is another broad ethical principle underlying caregiving.

Ethical Guidelines for Action

- If you have cause to think that your patient is likely to accuse you of improper or immoral conduct, *keep a careful documentary log* of what was said and done, how you responded, the date, time, witnesses, and circumstances of the event. You might include your interpretations of the event in a special section. The

ethical principles and motives that guided your action should be included also. Taking these steps is especially important with aggressive or paranoidal (suspicious and accusatory) patients. The goals are to give you peace of mind, to protect your image as a responsible caregiver, and to give you a strong legal defense if you should be accused of improper conduct.
- If you have doubts or ethical questions about a caregiving procedure, *consult with experts* at long-term care facilities, hospitals, or university social work departments. *Confer with friends* who are also caregivers. Use their consensus, combined with your considered judgment, as a guide.

Belonging to a Community

Spirituality includes belonging to a community. A community is a group of people bound together by common purposes and values. They take responsibility for one another's welfare. Love is the glue that holds a community together—a love characterized by nondemanding and uncritical acceptance of the other person, along with a commitment to the welfare of all members.

Community can include extended family, neighborhood, village, religious congregation, or stranger groups with common values such as the commitment to seek truth and provide mutual support. Community can be viewed in a global sense also, because we are one human race bound together by common needs for survival. Community offers continuity and a historical dimension to life.

One of the greatest concerns of older people is that when they die they will be forgotten. What is going to help you reduce this concern, not only in your patients but also as far as your being remembered for your contributions? It will be your community of concerned neighbors.

What this spiritual dimension of community means for you as a caregiver is that you can feel confident that you belong to a significant group that offers identity and support now and reentry opportunities later when your caregiving tasks cease.

Guidelines for Community

- If you enjoy writing, keep a short journal of your caregiving experiences to give you the feeling of continuity and provide a legacy. It will have emotional satisfactions also.
- Keep or establish your roots in your local community. One of the most painful results of isolation in the caregiver role is a feeling of loneliness and abandonment.
- Reach out to a religious community. If you do not have an affiliation, explore your options. Most churches, synagogues, and mosques have outreach ministries that offer much-needed emotional support for isolated caregivers.
- Join a support group. You can find these groups to meet your special needs for dementia, stroke, Parkinson's, or cancer patients in your care.

Values

The easiest way to describe values is to ask, "What do you hold dear?" "Who is important to you and why?" Values include sayings that have guided your life. For example, when someone hurts you, you recall biblical verses such as, "Put away from you all bitterness, wrath and anger," and, "Turn the other cheek." Others from family tradition or readings serve as value guides. Examples are: "Life is a bowl of cherries"; "Suffering is virtuous and moulds character"; "A cheerful heart is a gift from God"; "Hope springs eternal in the human breast"; and "Every day in every way I am getting better and better."

Some values are contradictory, such as saying, on the one hand, "Beat the other person down before he can do it to you." This value conflicts with its opposite: "Look out for the other person's welfare first; forgive him or her and put your needs aside." How do you handle this conflict between self-interest and the welfare of others in your life?

Service

One of a caregiver's greatest spiritual needs is to affirm the meaning and value of service to others. To serve our patients is the deepest expression of the Spirit working in our lives. It opens rather than closes us. Service can be a source of daily satisfaction and ultimate life fulfillment that goes far beyond material or achievement definitions of success. Albert Schweitzer, the great humanitarian who served as a healer in the jungles of Africa, said that the only folks who will be really happy are those who have sought and found how to serve. The Islamic prophet, Muhammad, said also that a man's true wealth is the good he does in the world. Service generates a healing force that accumulates one-by-one to the healing of the entire world. What are your values about service?

Love

We assert that love is the basic value underlying all caregiving services. Love is one of those supreme human feelings that is difficult to define in words but is recognized by all humans as the ultimate essential human experience.

We understand love best when we lose it. We do not presume to do justice to this important topic so briefly here, but we offer a few statements of others to stimulate your thinking about the meaning of love:

- Love is ultimate caring.
- Love is letting go of fear.
- Love is the expression of God.
- Love is unconditional.
- Love is our only reality.
- Love is feeling good about ourselves and others.
- Love is the basis for inner peace.
- Love is the blood of life, the power of the reunion in the separated.
- Mother love is our earliest lesson.
- Mature love: I am loved because I love.
- Love is the bridge over separation.

The word *love* is used commonly to describe motivation for unselfish, caring service to others, as in the phrases *a labor of love* and *brotherly love*. What does love mean to you, personally and in your role as a caregiver? Do you think it is possible to love your care receiver and, at the same time, resent him or her for imposing on your life? Are you aware of your simultaneous feelings of love and resentment toward your care receiver? Such mixed feelings are common experiences of caregivers.

Guidelines for Using Values

- *Leave a spiritual legacy* for your family, citing the values that guided your life, such as, "It was important to me when the going got rough to keep slogging ahead until the task was finished"; "I grew up with the idea that nothing was to be wasted"; "I remember that old saying that cleanliness is next to godliness"; or, "Happiness depends on the way you look at things, not the way they really are." In Jewish culture, the *ethical will* is a collection of value statements left for descendants. If caregivers followed this practice, such a will would include your fondest wishes and your choicest blessings that you wished to convey to your survivors. Such a legacy could strengthen your resolve to share your life and to specify how you want to be remembered. The act of making this ethical legacy could also enrich your present life and make your caregiving tasks more tolerable and rewarding.

- *Listen to the stories of your care receiver* (which you have probably heard many times), but listen this time for the spiritual history and values imbedded in those stories. Make a mental lifeline for the events and use them as a takeoff point for discussions at your care receiver's level of understanding. For example, as a starter you might say something like, "Your childhood seemed to be a happy time for you, but your adult life had one sad loss after another"; "What struck me so forcefully in your descriptions of those sad events were the threads of hope and optimism that wound through them"; "Those threads sort of wrapped your life together so you could go on"; or, "Did you see it that way, too, or did you see something different?" Note that the use of an image, "threads," makes the discussion more concrete and understandable for a person with limited residual mental capacity. Note also that after you give your impressions of your patient's stories, you ask for confirmation from him or her, such as, "Am I correct?" Asking the question also gives you a hint about whether or not your care receiver understood your summary of their story.

Beliefs

Beliefs are statements we assume to be true or useful, such as, "I believe in the healing power of prayer," or, "I believe that love is the greatest force in the world," or "I believe in a higher power—an ultimate power, God," or, "I believe that I am becoming a better person every day." Beliefs provide guiding principles for everyday living. These beliefs, when stated clearly and systematically, are a great source of hope, comfort, and self-worth. They provide a sense of direction and personal identity. We are what we believe!

When beliefs become fixed and formalized they become doctrines. Doctrines, especially when claimed to be divinely inspired, become essential foundations for religions; religions need institutions such as churches, mosques, and synagogues. Have you, as a caregiver, clarified your relationship to formalized religion? It may be helpful to realize that you can be spiritual without being religious; conversely, you can be religious without being spiritual. You might not like this kind of split; if so, how do you integrate or differentiate spirituality and religiosity?

Your Sense of Humor

Value of Humor

Caregiving has its rewards, including some momentary pleasures. However, many caregivers perceive it as a grim existence. This section aims to lighten your sense of burden and bring more joy into your life.

Laughter is healing. It maintains our general state of wellness, reduces muscle tension, stimulates stress-reducing hormones, and strengthens the immune system. During laughter there is increasing oxygen in the blood, and while blood pressure rises during the laughter, it subsides considerably afterward. Marilyn Grey, a stress management consultant, claims we need twenty laughs a day to stay healthy (the average is only two).[3] Our problem as adults is that we have lost our childhood ability to laugh at anything. Witness the four-year-old who says, "Watch me burp," and then laughs uproariously.

Grey said, "Laughter is the magic that lifts us on joyful wings and beyond pain and despair. Laughter is a miracle."[4] For example, when you feel everything is going wrong and wonder why you are singled out for those caregiving hassles, you might conjure up some humor for the situation.

Laughter can shift attention from the boredom and pain of your caregiving tasks to the pleasant side of caregiving and tension release. Laughter also can bond two former strangers. Victor Borge, the musical humorist, said that laughter is the shortest distance between two people. Humor can defuse a tense situation arising between you and your patient. It is difficult to be angry when you have had a good laugh together.

Developing a Sense of Humor

You are thinking, perhaps, that trying to laugh or even the humor in your painful situation is just not realistic. You see your never-ending, totally absorbing caregiving tasks. You also probably think that you just do not have the time or inclination to explore the possible humor in your caregiving situation. Maybe you say that you do not have a sense of humor. We urge you to try, even though it might be difficult and awkward at first. It is worth the extra effort because the benefits are so great.

Having a sense of humor can be learned. There are several ways to perceive the humor in everyday situations, especially in serious, absurd, and painful caregiving situations. Caregivers in our study reported consistently that exhaustion was the primary enemy of humor. You will find something useful to try in the following "laundry list" of suggestions.

Suggestions for Finding Humor

- Seek at least one experience a day around which to have a deep belly laugh. Call a friend to ask if he or she has had an experience that you could both chuckle over (an absurd or exaggerated situation, an incongruous event, a joke, a cartoon).
- Borrow or purchase a collection of video- or audio-tapes on humor or a recorded program by Jack Benny or Milton Berle, for example.
- Find a TV sitcom you enjoy, or tune into *America's Funniest Home Videos*. Laugh with the audience and soon you will be laughing spontaneously.
- Remind yourself that the world is absurd, but that it works out all right and, in time, makes sense. Wander through the absurdity until you come out on top. To the comedian, nothing in life makes sense. For example, W. C. Fields, the lovable comic of years back, was buffeted by many tragic events; however, he had a humorous way of kicking back at the world. Thus, he was able to rise above the sadness and injustices in his life. For Joan Rivers, a contemporary comedienne, all of life is absurd.
- To help see the absurdities in your life, watch films or tapes of the masters of comedy on the American

scene: Jonathan Winters, W. C. Fields, Red Skelton, Richard Pryor, George Carlin, Bob Newhart, Jack Benny, Irma Bombeck, Robin Williams, Milton Berle, Don Adams, Peter Sellers, George Burns, Jackie Gleason, Billy Crystal, Sid Caesar, Woody Allen, Johnny Carson, George Gobel, Jack Lemmon, Walter Mathau, and many contemporary humorists. The laughter these comedians evoke helps to diffuse tense and painful situations. When you have had a long, frustrating, and exhausting day, for example, seeing these comedians' exaggerated, slapstick behavior, outrageous statements, convoluted predicaments, and efforts to make sense of life helps to relieve your tensions. It also reaffirms the fact that your life may not be so bad after all. When you feel sorry for yourself, Red Skelton's antics as Freddie the Freeloader will help to get back on track. Some experimenting may be required before you see the parallels to your life or until they really tickle you.

- You cannot remain on a downer very long when you hear Woody Allen play his neurotic role and complain that "part of my problem is that I'm a sex object." Similarly, Peter Sellers, in the Pink Panther movies tries to be a good cop, but nothing works right for him. One goal of all comedians is to alleviate suffering, so we suggest that you find that pearl of amusement and relief when they inflate life beyond its normal size with their outrageous behavior. Norman Cousins, former editor of *Saturday Review*, healed himself of a serious degenerative disease by watching funny films and laughing throughout the day.[5]
- Watch a film of slapstick comedians with the expectation that their crazy antics will bring out a good belly laugh. Clowns have done this for centuries. Some examples from American culture are Laurel and Hardy, Charlie Chaplin, Victor Borge, the Marx

Brothers, Lilly Tomlin, and the Helzapoppin group. If you are not familiar with American humorists, pick some from your own cultural tradition.
- Tell a story on yourself about an incident that was humiliating or embarrassingly funny. Self-putdowns help to see the humility and humanity in tragic situations. Phyllis Diller said that if all of life were beautiful there would be no comedy. As awful as things may be, we see through humor that life goes on. Life would be intolerable if we did not have humor. So, your assignment is to find the gems of humor in your everyday life. Humor helps to fix those bad days.
- Get into a playful mood. Take a deep breath and just spontaneously laugh uproariously as if you were happy or the situation is laughable. This act of deception tricks the body into thinking that the situation is funny. Many actors do this in preparing for their roles. They act; then they feel the emotion from their actions. So—sing, dance, and act happy to feel happy!
- Sing a song with a smile when you feel out of sorts. Remember Anna in *The King and I* when her son asked her if she was afraid? She replied in song, "Whenever I feel afraid, I whistle a happy tune."
- It would be well to avoid so-called *black humor* or *gallows humor*. While intended to shock us and challenge our thinking, it often backfires and offends. Examples are gross racial and ethnic jokes, gender or age ridicule, and jokes about death and suffering. These efforts are likely to increase distress. In our opinion, it is preferable to stick with the light humor described above.
- Learn to tell jokes. Yes, you may have difficulty remembering the punch lines, but practice until you have two or three in your repertoire. They will trigger memories in other folks, and off you go!

Your Inner Journey

You have explored some essential resources for your self-care. You have confronted your definition of spirituality. You have examined also some dimensions of spirituality that we suggested—morals and ethics, beliefs, and values, meaning, and community.

You explored the possibility of rediscovering the child within you—that joyful, spontaneous, impish, mirthful creature. Even though your caregiving tasks leave you with a grim outlook, we hope our suggestions for adding some pleasure and laughter to your life will ease your burden.

In the next chapter we will explore other facets of your inner life—how to cope with your problems of diminished and lost intimacy.

Notes

1. Joseph Campbell, *The Hero with a Thousand Faces* (Cleveland: World, 1949).
2. Abraham Maslow, *Toward a Psychology of Being* (Princeton: D. Van Nostrand, 1972).
3. Marilyn Grey, "Laughter as a Tool in Stress Management," speech presented at the Seventh Annual Northwest Wellness Conference for Seniors, Seaside, Oregon, October 1996.
4. Marilyn Grey, *It's All in Your Head* (Lynnwood, WA: Greymatter, 1995).
5. Norman Cousins, *Head First* (New York: E. P. Dutton, 1989).

4
The Quest for Intimacy

Trying for intimacy and open communication is a continual battle, one that I am losing fast.

—Sue, a caregiver

When Intimacy Fades

One of the great losses experienced by caregivers, spouses particularly, is the reduction or disappearance of shared intimate relationships. The majority of spousal caregivers we interviewed described this loss of intimacy—along with their loneliness and sexual frustration—in poignant terms. **Sue's** lament (as quoted above) is typical. She went on to say, "I mourn for what we used to have, and long to have it again. We can't talk anymore. I am lonely and frustrated." **Laura** said also, "The loss of communication with a spouse can be devastating. The need for close human contact such as caressing, simple touching, seeing, hearing, are essential parts of the sex drive. This need is at no time greater than in old age, when reassurance that someone cares is appreciated. When this is no longer possible, relief can come through self-gratification." Laura's reaction emphasizes the painful loneliness, reduced communication, grasping at alternatives, and lack of demonstrative appreciation that accompany the lost intimacy.

Intimacy in the context of this chapter refers primarily to caressing, fondling, and intercourse, although intimate feelings can be manifested also through endearing words, hugs, gentle touch, playful cuddles, and holding hands. Intimate feelings of love can be communicated also through warm, steady, affirming eye contact.

This chapter describes the problems caregivers face with these losses of intimacy. In addition, we offer the following options: (1) remain celibate; (2) engage in a sexual affair; (3) engage in self-gratification; (4) sublimate needs for intimacy with activity; and (5) explore same-sex relationships. We are not advocating any particular option.

We have cited these examples to assure you who are currently giving care that you are not alone in your frustration and loneliness. You can be assured also from these and later examples that you have great inner strengths and sensual resources to draw upon. You who are prospective caregivers can get a glimpse of personal conflicts likely to be experienced in efforts to satisfy your needs for intimacy and communication. William Masters, a sex therapist, tells this story: "Recently we had a lovely lady bring her husband in for therapy. He was 72 and had been impotent for three years. She said she wanted us to help him. 'because I don't have too much time and I don't want to waste it.' She was 82."

Are Your Sexual Attitudes Showing?

Regardless of the options a caregiver chooses for fulfilling intimacy needs, attitudes about body functions, seeking pleasure, and intimate body contact help or hinder fulfillment. A first step for caregivers desiring to improve their intimate lives would be to do some soul-searching about their attitudes toward sexuality. Honest self-confrontation about traditional attitudes of dominance, exploitation, neglect, or abuse would be an essential first step to changing them. Let us look at some of the negative attitudes that could interfere with intimacy.

Coping with Negative Attitudes

Viewing sexual activity and the body as dirty or sinful is a key obstacle to intimacy. Granted that there are sexual acts that are an affront to sensitive and caring people, do you believe that these actions can be avoided without condemning the entire spectrum of sexual behaviors?

Repressive attitudes were common at certain times in history, just as free expression characterized other times. For example, on one hand, the repression of sexuality in the turn-of-the-century Victorian era represents one extreme. It still has its faithful adherents. On the other hand, Eastern Tantric exercises of ancient times involved ritual sexual pleasures that are still used to achieve spiritual transcendence in some cultures. The sexual pleasures outlined in the ancient Kama Sutra of Vatsayana is another example of pleasures often associated with spiritual rituals. The classical Greeks put erotic pleasures high on their list of the good things of life.

The point here is that your cultural conditioning is the main determiner of your attitudes about intimate pleasures. The key to change is confronting these repressive attitudes from your past culture, religious injunctions, and family rules. Then make a decision whether or not to deny their hold on your present intimate life. What strict rules of conduct were part of your moral education, such as: no masturbation, no nudity, no sex outside of marriage, and no homosexual acts? Did violations of these past injunctions generate guilt? How do you view the changing mores involving sexual freedom? Where do you stand on this issue of repression/expression? What negative attitudes and rules about intimate behavior govern your present activities? Do you want to change them?

Encourage Positive Attitudes about Intimacy

The second step toward satisfactory intimacy is becoming more aware of positive attitudes toward human nudity and intimate acts. Some views that make the choices about intimacy easier are that bodily pleasures are acceptable and that they are not decadent or sinful except as you believe them to be so. A key prior question is whether any of these behaviors do damage physically or psychologically to you or to others. A positive attitude in this connection is to say to one's self, *I am a responsible person. I act in my best interest, and that of the other person and of society.*

A cluster of positive attitudes facilitate easy and responsible intimacy. Examples are: "The human body is a beautiful creation of God"; "Sex is a divine gift"; "Sexual activity is a sacred, creative act"; and "Intimate activity is a spiritual experience (loving, caring, cherishing, respecting, for example)." One of the exciting developments in the present study of human relations is the integration of sex and spirit. It has been said that sex is the path to the soul. It is an ancient idea that optimal sex is the fusion of spiritual energy with sexual energy; however, we need to rediscover it periodically and redefine it in modern, personal terms.

What Are Your Choices?

When you are more aware and feel comfortable with your negative and positive attitudes about intimacy, it is time to make some decisions. The difficult dilemmas of choice for the spousal caregiver are clear. We suggest you review the following options with an open mind. Then give yourself some self-confrontive counseling and weigh the pros and cons of each choice, including not making a choice.

Take a deep breath and decide. Feel right about your choice, even though you will probably feel uneasy about it for a while. We do not recommend any specific option. We are all so different in backgrounds, needs, and attitudes that each of us must make these delicate decisions for ourselves.

Remain Celibate

This means accepting the restrictions on intimacy imposed by your current caregiving tasks. You could view this restriction as an unfortunate happenstance, a quirk of fate, or part of a divine plan. Thus, you would give up immediate plans for pursuing outlets for intimacy, except for the occasional hugs and kisses from relatives and friends. We sense that the majority of caregivers decide this way, at least temporarily.

This choice to remain celibate and to disavow intimacy needs requires some strong denial. You must tell yourself that giving and receiving intimacies is not important at this time. If you have strong moral restraints, you tell yourself also that you wish to remain faithful to your marital vows regardless of your own needs. The ultimate self-message, however, is to tell yourself that caregiving is a special ministry that takes precedence over all other choices. This choice is illustrated by one of our caregivers, who said, "Caregiving is my mission in life at the present time. It is a special ministry. I will do my best for myself and the person in my care."

The choice of celibacy need not be limited to a fleeting hug from friends and relatives. A planned effort to increase touching opportunities is essential to personal well-being. To deny the rewards of touch is to thwart a primal human sensory need. The skin is a very sensitive organ, with millions of receptors.

Positive touch releases nourishing brain chemicals that have good health effects. Examples are reduced blood pressure, a lowered heart rate, and improved immune function. Every mother knows the soothing and health-producing effects of gentle touch on the infant. Numerous studies of infant massage over the years have shown that such infants' mood improves, they sleep better, and the premies leave the hospital earlier. Studies of older adults, similarly, indicate the values of touch and massage in particular for improved health and well-being. There are many positive side effects for the caregivers who do the touching also.

Touch deprivation is a common characteristic of the nontactile U.S. society. We are very cautious about touching because we think it may lead inexorably to unwanted sexual intimacy. It is unfortunate that the harassing touch of a few unethical people has led to even tighter social and legal restrictions. On the other hand, there are numerous cultures where public touch in the form of hugging, embracing, and hand holding is common and accepted.

So, you are saying, "Yes, I agree that touch has all these good effects, but I do not have the opportunity for even a hand touch from anyone." We realize how frustrating such a situation can be, but we encourage you to develop an intentional program to increase your touching opportunities.

The first step is to examine your attitudes about touch. Are they open and accepting, or do you tend to tighten up when close? Do your attitudes toward others, and your facial expressions say, *Keep your distance*, or do they encourage a touch or a hug? You may need some feedback from friends on this communication point.

Some people appear to be natural huggers. Hugging is very acceptable in some social groups, but it must be exercised very discreetly so as not to be misunderstood as seduction. Among friends and relatives it usually is accepted, but one person must take the initiative. Is it to be you?

Perhaps you will need to learn to be more comfortable in such a social role. If hugging seems too brazen to you, perhaps a light hand touch or prolonged handshake would be a comfortable starter.

A professional massage is a way to fulfill this need for contact as well as obtain the health and relaxation benefits. Even back and neck rubs from friends and associates are helpful if your attitude is accepting. Giving such massages to friends and, of course, to your care receiver is a way of obtaining additional feelings of well-being.

If you have not had a professional massage, we strongly recommend that you try it during one of your respite periods. Massages last for one-half to one hour and come in different styles, from deep muscle pressure to sweeping surface hand movements. Professionals are licensed and operate very ethically. It is unfortunate that massage has acquired a cloudy reputation because it sometimes is associated with prostitution. A good reference should help to avoid such "massage parlors."

You may want to consider some of the preceding suggestions to make your choice of celibacy more tolerable. They also will help to avoid the anxiety of the choices described below. We do not assume that some form of intimacy satisfaction is essential to being a good caregiver. Many caregivers appear to get along just fine, especially if they are skilled at giving themselves constructive self-messages that it is OK if they do not have intimate sensory satisfactions.

Engage in a Sexual Affair

Those caregivers who choose the option of an outside sexual outlet often appear to pay a heavy price. Such a venture requires great expenditure of energy to repress the likely guilt and fear. One of our caregivers, for example, feared the price would be too high: "We are entitled to have a sexual and emotional relationship, but I, for one, could never live with the guilt and feeling of betrayal of my values that would accompany it."

Other caregivers decide that the price is worth it. Let us hear from some of them: "As caretakers we owe it to ourselves to have some happiness and feel no guilt. I miss so many things about my spouse, but the lover is the greatest loss." Another said, "I find the impotence and his lack of concern for any of my needs much harder burdens to bear than the physical illness. I love him very much; it hurts sometimes to be rejected so often. I am considering alternatives for me." One caregiver from the Well Spouse Foundation Survey said, "I miss sexual contact very much. But more than that is the profound and pervading sadness and grief at the loss of friendship and shared intimacy. When sex became a painful reminder of the losses, it was abandoned. But I have to survive, too. I think a discreet affair is not a sin, but is life-saving. I had one and it was good for both of us. The guilt was severe. It is not an easy answer." Another said, "We've discussed my having an affair and of course it makes him sad, but he said if I have to, I have to. His main fear is that it will eventually lead to my leaving him. I bear his physical problems. If I bore my emotional problems alone, I would only resent it and him."[1]

If you have decided to try this option, the first step would be constructing an elaborate chain of rationalizations to have the affair. The caregivers cited previously offer some reasons for their anticipated affairs. Additional examples of such rationalizations are: *It is my turn to have some pleasure; I have earned it; It is physically and psychologically healthier to have an active sex life than to repress and deny my intimate needs;* and *sexual activity is needed to keep the sex drive alive and functional.* You probably can think of more reasons to justify your choice.

Additional positive self-messages are important to support a decision to have an affair: *I need not feel guilty or ashamed; I have considered the alternatives and the consequences for all concerned; I am willing to risk those short- and long-term consequences (emotional, health, legal, and familial); I will be responsible for any choice I make;* and *I feel good about myself.*

Once you have decided to start a new intimate relationship, it is essential that you feel comfortable with your choice. It is also important to take all the precautions necessary to protect your health and welfare.

Engage in Self-Gratification

Self-gratification and *self-pleasuring* are contemporary terms for masturbation. It is an attractive choice for many caregivers as a substitute for a former relationship with a partner. While not as emotionally consequential or complex as an affair, this choice poses strong resistance for some caregivers. Since you may have grown up in a family with strong religious prohibitions against self-pleasuring, you may feel sinful and guilty for choosing this option. Remember, it was only a few years ago that the term for masturbation was *self-abuse*. Parents used drastic predictions about going blind or insane to control what they regarded as reprehensible and sinful behavior.

There are many individual reactions to this polarizing issue about whether or not to engage in self-gratification. Some are unequivocally opposed to the practice. One caregiver in our survey said, "I think that masturbation is shameful and abnormal." Another, with a favorable experience, said, "Masturbation, rather than being painfully improper, can be viewed simply as an alternative sexual experience." Some try it and are disillusioned, as one caregiver in the Well Spouse Survey reported: "I try to get sensual pleasure in other ways, such as in self-pleasuring, but it does not fill the void. There is fear of losing that sexual part of me."

The current social climate appears to be generally accepting of self-gratification, especially for situations where there is no satisfactory sexual partner available. Those who favor self-pleasuring as a way of fulfilling their needs look upon it as a positive and creative spiritual experience. Some view it as an antidote to loneliness.

All of these views suggest that a first step in considering self-pleasuring is becoming fully aware of your own attitudes toward masturbation and bodily pleasures in general. Let your inner spirit be your guide. The principal issue for caregivers is whether or not this is the best choice for themselves at this time. Feeling a sense of rightness about the decision is essential. Thus, there would be no need for guilt, shame, or lowered self-esteem to complicate an already-difficult choice.

Sublimate Needs for Intimacy with Activity

This choice assumes that a rigorous activity program can reduce the need for intimacy. This choice is based on the underlying psychological theory that tensions generated in one domain (sexual drive) can be reduced by activity in another domain (such as social activities). While usually not a long-term solution, busying yourself in activities such as sports, socializing, hobbies, music, or satisfying work can be temporarily distracting.

We hear you saying, "Yes, but where do I find the time to do anything but the demanding tasks of caregiving? Besides, my life is complicated by a painful loneliness. I just don't see many people anymore." This comment is probably short comfort, but immersing yourself in the demanding daily activities of caregiving such as lifting and supporting is a kind of sublimation. Some additional examples of sublimation activities are cleaning house, shopping, taking walks, and participating in an in-house exercise program.

Explore Same-Sex Relationships

Another option for coping with deprivation of intimacy is to seek comfort and fulfillment with a friend of the same sex. Even if gay or lesbian relationships are not acceptable to you, a close nonsexual relationship may be fulfilling. Maggie Kuhn, a respected authority on older-adult issues, makes a case for exploring the gay or lesbian route to intimacy for older deprived caregivers. For women, she cites greater availability of partners, more comfort, less complication and demand than heterosexual relationships, and equal or greater satisfaction.[2]

As in the options cited previously, this choice requires intensive awareness of your own attitudes toward same-sex relationships. It is a difficult choice because of the long condemnation of this activity in Western religious and medical traditions. A further complication is the current controversy about the extent to which homosexuality is genetic and the extent to which it is culturally induced. A decision would require more intensive research on this issue than we could provide in this brief exploration. In any case, there is much more social acceptance of this choice and increasing attention to problems of discrimination and violence against gay and lesbian people.

A Final Word

None of the solutions described in this chapter is easy. The choices are complicated and sometimes agonizing, but we hope that the options we have described here will make a little easier the decision of what to do with your intimacy needs. In summary, if intimacy is a problem, let us reassure you that whatever choice you make, it is important to maintain a conviction of rightness about your decision. Whatever decision you make, there probably will be occasional future second thoughts about it. Therefore, if you maintain this conviction and it appears prudent to consider changing your first choice, you can do so without stress. Talk it over with a trusted friend or counselor. Then act with confidence.

In the next chapter we will discuss how to make your life as a caregiver easier through more effective problem solving and smoother communication.

Notes

1. Deborah Hayden, "Forum: Sexuality and the Well Spouse," *Well Spouse Foundation Newsletter* 44 (November/December): 3 (888 Eighth Avenue, New York, NY, 10019).
2. Maggie Kuhn, *Maggie Kuhn on Aging* (Philadelphia: Westminster Press, 1977).

Recommended Reading

Aneshensel, Carol, et al. *Profiles in Caregiving: The Unexpected Cares*. San Diego: Academic Press, 1996.

5
How to Make Your Life Easier

One form of unconsciousness supports the survival self. Another supports the spiritual self. Problems arise when one crowds out the other.
—Arthur Deikman, psychiatrist

We hear caregivers saying repeatedly that "if you could help make my life easier and simpler, I would be very grateful." This chapter will tell you how to solve knotty problems more efficiently. In addition, since communication breakdowns make your life miserable at times, we will describe how to improve communication with the person in your charge. Your life will not only be easier, but it will also be much richer.

Problem Solving

Wouldn't it be wonderful if you could solve all your problems easily and effectively? Problem-solving effectiveness means having a variety of methods for solving personal problems. When you finish this chapter you will be able to apply three basic problem-solving strategies.

What kinds of problems are we talking about? Examples are: How and when should I consider moving my spouse to a nursing facility? How can I reach my care receiver, who is so mentally distant? What will I do when I "retire" from my present caregiving responsibility? How are we going to pay the rent this month? Where can I find respite services and how can I pay for them? How can I acquire more coping skills so I can make it through another month? What am I going to do with my rebellious teenager? Shall I keep my regular job or quit to take the pressure off while I'm a caregiver?

Trial and Error

Trial and error is the most common method of solving personal problems. You start with awareness of a situation that you wish would be different, such as *I want to communicate better with my care receiver*. Then you draw upon your experience and common sense, trying various approaches to find one that works. In this example, you would start by trying to talk with him or her directly, but quietly, with simple words. You might choose early morning, when your receiver is rested, fed, and relaxed. If this does not work, you might try a firmer and more authoritative tone. You might try this approach at a time when your receiver is in a mellow mood or when you are mirthful and teasing. The point is that you would try different ways of reaching your care receiver, based on your experience with him or her. Sometimes you use your experience combined with blind trial and error to reach for a solution. We jokingly call this approach the *muddling through* style. The clearest example is solving a cube puzzle. You press squares and rotate them until you stumble upon the solution. Then, next time you can solve the cube puzzle faster because of your tryout experience.

Summary of Steps in Trial-and-Error Problem Solving (Learning by Experience)

- Scan your experience and ask others for advice on possible solutions to your problem.

- Try them, starting with the most feasible. If it does not work, try another and another until you find a solution. (Remember the cube puzzle?)

Logical Problem Solving

This style is systematic and uses relevant information and logic. It is difficult to apply a purely logical approach to human problems because usually they are so complicated and the problems come in multiples—not simply one at a time. Take the problem, for example, of whether or not to put Grandpa in a long-term intensive-care facility. You could approach the question with logic that: his capacity for independent living has deteriorated, you are at the end of your patience, you cannot give him the level of care that he needs, and he could qualify for Medicaid. With the logical approach, you also might consider alternatives such as group homes, bringing a chore worker into your home, and changing family caregivers. You gather as much information about the problem as you can.

In logical problem solving you trying to minimize impulsive feeling-directed solutions. When the final logical decisions are made, however, they usually come down to how the proposed solution feels: Does the proposed solution feel right in light of all the facts?

For problems requiring special information and certainty of outcomes, the logical approach serves you best. Examples of such problems are buying a new home and the preceding example—deciding whether to put Grandpa in a nursing facility. There are sequential steps that you follow in logical and unemotional fashion.

Steps in Logical Problem Solving

1. *Become aware that a problem exists.* Recall the example used previously regarding the family's perceived

need to place Grandpa in a long-term intensive-care program. His behavior is annoying and stressful for his caregiver and her family. It is important at this step to develop a *problem set*. This means getting a realistic grasp of the facts in the problem situation. You, the caregiver, "own" the problem because you are the principal person affected. Gramps probably does not think **he** has a problem.

2. *State the Problem.* A clearly stated problem looks like a goal. The statement contrasts where you are now—confused, annoyed, anxious, and stressed—with where you want to be. The temptation to jump impulsively from step 1 to a solution is avoided by answering the question: "What is the real problem?" In the example of Grandpa, the problem is his uncontrollable tendencies to wander and get lost, coupled with his inability to take care of himself. So, a clear problem statement would be: "Grandpa's wandering tendencies and inability to care for himself cause us sufficient concern and stress to get more supervision for him." This statement describes the kind of problem (uncontrolled behavior), who is affected (the caregiver and the family), who is causing it (Grandpa), and what the goal is (more intensive supervision). Note that the caregiver did not jump to the conclusion that a long-term care facility was necessarily the best solution to this problem.

3. *Formulate a goal.* After thinking through the clear problem statement, it is time to change it to a goal statement. The goal is to "develop a plan for more intensive, round-the-clock supervision for Grandpa."

4. *Develop alternatives.* You, the caregiver who owns the problem, sit down with your family, support network members, or professional consultants to:

(a) describe the problem and the goal, and (b) generate alternative plans to reach your goal. Some goals that you might discover in your brainstorming, for example, are more assistance with supervision from your family, financing for a group home to give twenty-four hour supervision, finding a suitable respite center, or long-term placement in a nursing home. This step obviously requires research into sources of information for solving the problem.

5. *Decide among alternative plans.* After identifying all the various ways to extend supervision for Grandpa, you choose the one that looks most feasible now. Suppose it is a nearby group home. Before taking action, do an analysis of the pros and cons of this choice. Draw a vertical line down the middle of a sheet of paper. On the left side list all the things you can think of that are favorable toward this choice, such as proximity. On the right side, list all the ideas that would be against your choice, such as financial. Usually in this pro and con thinking process, the feasibility of a particular choice becomes apparent. Let us assume that your analysis confirms the choice of a group home. It is close, it is small, it is financially feasible, and Grandpa would have companions there. Now you are ready to move from planning to action.

6. *Try out and evaluate the alternative.* So, you place Grandpa in this home after proper orientation and preparation. It is understood that this is a trial placement to see how it goes. You find after two weeks that Grandpa is adjusting well to his new environment, so you decide to continue the placement, with Grandpa making periodic visits to your home.

You undoubtedly have solved problems with similar steps many times, but try on this process to see if you are solving problems effectively at this time. You will observe that this logical process may appear laborious, but it prevents hasty solutions. Vaguely defined problems just beg for fast solutions. Furthermore, while thinking through the logic of this problem-solving process and trying to get more precision in defining the problem it is easier to keep emotions under control. Finally, this style of solving problems does not leave you with an irrevocable decision. You can think in terms of provisional tryouts while you gather more information about the long-term suitability of your choice.

Summary of Steps for Logical Problem Solving

- State the problem.
- Change the problem to a goal.
- Generate possible alternative solutions.
- Collect information on the alternative solutions.
- Select the best-appearing alternative.
- Try out the alternative.
- Evaluate the solution.
- Try another alternative solution if necessary.

Application of Logical Problem Solving to Caregiving

Recall a past problem you have faced. What steps did you go through? How effective was your effort? How was it similar to or different from the process described previously?

Choose a current caregiving problem—a situation that you do not like and wish that it would be different. Choose a problem without a readily apparent solution, such as the one faced by **Delia**. She is a caregiver for an eight-year-old neurologically impaired son, her only child. Until now,

Delia has provided most of his care. She receives some help, reluctantly, from her second husband.

Delia's eight years of caregiving have taken a heavy physical and emotional toll, so she feels she cannot continue with the present arrangement. Her husband, who works full-time, is unwilling to increase his part in the care. Delia would like to go back to work, but she knows that her pay would not be enough to cover a full-time professional caregiver. What is her basic problem? What are the subproblems she needs to solve?

What is her main goal—to reduce her burden, to find help, to go back to work, to get her husband to take more responsibility? Which of these are subgoals?

What difficulties did you have? Was the logical method appropriate for your problem? What did you learn about your problem-solving style? Was this problem too complex to find an early or easy solution? Does the problem need division into subproblems? The style of problem solving must fit the type of problem—in this case, well-defined problems.

Intuitive and Creative Styles of Problem Solving

Characteristics of Intuitive Thinking

You certainly have had intuitions about solutions to past problems. The basic issue for caregivers is: How much can I trust my intuitions? Our answer is that most of us do not trust our intuitions enough. More answers are presented later in this chapter.

Intuitions are based on vague bodily sensations combined with hunches based partly on logic. Intuitions are ways of knowing without knowing how you know. Sometimes they appear to be risky leaps into the unknown, so intuitions are considered by some people to be mystical or disreputable. In many cultures, intuition is the preferred method for making decisions. So, try the intuitive method yourself if you have not done so in the past.

Steps in Intuitive Problem Solving

1. *Receptivity*. An essential mental set for intuitive solutions is the caregiver's openness to new ideas and nonrigid thought. Novel and unconventional thinking are prized. Patience and submissiveness are virtues, because the more aggressively you search for solutions, the more elusive they tend to become. Having a large background of facts in the problem area helps, because a basic condition for intuitive problem solvers is to be saturated with the subject. This is somewhat contradictory, since having too much experience and factual background is often used as a rationalization for staying in the mental rut and not seeing the creative possibilities in novel solutions.
2. *Asking questions*. A preparatory step is asking many questions from different perspectives. Solutions often are limited by the way you ask the questions. Usually, after you have asked many questions and mulled over the problem (called *incubation*), a solution often appears in your awareness. Relaxed concentration on the problem and visualization of how it appears in the present and might look in the future facilitate solving it.
3. Finally, you must trust your body wisdom, since solutions emerge from emotional data banks called *organismic wisdom*. To do this kind of intuitional thinking you must believe that most of what you need to know is already there, stored in your body.

The basic question is: How can you tap this organismic wisdom to solve your caregiving problem?

Conditions for Intuition

Intuitive problem solving does not have a fixed and linear set of steps as in the logical model. Some of the conditions and attitudes you must have to facilitate intuitive solutions are:

1. *A state of physical relaxation.* You must have a routine like the one we described in chapter 2 concerning stress management. The resulting relaxation encourages receptiveness and opens you to ideas, hunches, and extrasensory perceptions.
2. *Incubation time.* This is relaxed time for mulling over ideas, playing around with the problem in your fantasy, breaking it down into parts, and redefining it. It is a time for considering facts and inviting alternative solutions to pop into your awareness. It is time to be sure that the questions you are asking yourself are the important ones.

To someone watching you do this contemplative mulling it appears that not much is going on, but your thoughts are moving rapidly in many directions. A good way to illustrate this style is to examine Robert Pirsig's *Zen and the Art of Motorcycle Maintenance.* When his cycle stopped running he went into a receptive incubation state. He stared silently at the broken cycle for a long time. He asked questions from the viewpoint of the cycle and shed his old ideas on what might be wrong. He also avoided impulsive action that might have damaged the machine further. He "became" the cycle for a while and encouraged it to "tell him" what was wrong. He avoided rigid thinking about what the problem might be and was humbly open to new approaches.[1]

Intuitive thinking is not possible when the caregiver has rigid ideas about a desired solution. A dramatic illustration is the Indian monkey trapper. To capture monkeys alive and uninjured, the trapper cuts a hole in a coconut chained to a stake. The hole is a little smaller than a monkey's fist. He puts goodies in the coconut, and when the monkey grabs a handful he cannot get his hand out without releasing the goodies. While the monkey is engaged in this rigid thinking about his choices, the trapper pops a bag over his head.

Summary of Intuitive Problem Solving

- Allow for receptivity of novel and unconventional ideas.
- Ask questions.
- Assume a relaxed body state.
- Allow the answers to emerge from body awareness.
- Allow time to incubate ideas.
- Back away for a while and recycle the process if you get stuck.
- Look for the shift from tension to relaxation as a sign of approaching solution.

Experiential Focusing

This approach is closely related to the intuitive problem-solving method just described. It is a method of attending to the felt body experience of the problem.[2] It is a productive approach to use when the problem is vague, logical attempts to solve it have failed, or the solution appears to be elusive. There is a sequence of steps for the caregiver to follow that emphasizes awareness of the body. As in intuitive problem solving, the basic assumption is that the solutions to many of your vaguely defined problems lie in your bodily wisdom.

Steps in Experiential Focusing

1. Describe how you are experiencing your body now—relaxed, tense, restless, hot?
2. Describe your feelings about these sensations—joy, worry, anger, or dread, for example.
3, State your awareness about how your vague problem feels in your body. (Connect awareness from steps 1 and 2.)
4. Without pressing, you probably will experience a shift from the known part of the problem (your body sensations) to the unknown. To get to the unknown part of the problem, ask yourself what images or words flow forth to match your sensations, a process called *aboutness*. Receptiveness is important here also, because it is necessary to listen to, not talk to, your body. You need to do this several times with different images, until the aboutness results in a shift of body sensation from tenseness to relaxation and a great sense of release. The answer, or solution, feels right.

If this process of listening to the wisdom of your body does not help you toward a solution, then stop. Focus on the experience of being "stuck." Ask, *What is this body experience of being stuck, this frustration, saying to me? What additional questions do I need to ask myself? Am I aware of subtle changes in sensation (from tenseness to release)?* Sometimes it helps if you distance yourself from the process for a while. Come back to it later, but be alert in the meantime for images and feelings that indicate a shift in awareness of your body sensations. Images may appear to give hints of possible solutions.

Then try the process again until you get that feeling of rightness about the solution. For example, you might be considering moving to a smaller, one-floor residence to make care easier and more personal, but you have some doubts and fears. You have tried the logical methods of analyzing this problem with little satisfaction. Connecting body sensations to feelings and images helped to get a more clear assurance that going ahead with the change was the right thing to do. Again, you trusted your body's wisdom, and it felt right. But you also had checked out the reality considerations, such as higher costs and moving hassles, against lower taxes and lower utility bills.

The kind of decision just cited illustrates the use of several modes of problem solving in tandem—logical, intuitive, imagery, and trust of body messages. Remember, your goal is to develop problem-solving competence, which includes flexibility and the use of multiple strategies on a single caregiving problem.

Application of Intuitive Thinking to Caregiving

There are many lessons for caregiver survival from this discussion of intuition. Think of situations where you might have profitably used this intuitive style of problem solving. Were there incidents where your rigid thinking got you into difficulty? Think of situations where you could use Pirsig's motorcycle repair approach to a problem. Do you find it difficult to trust your body wisdom? At a simple level, does it tell you when it is tired and wants rest? At a more complex level, does your body give you a hint about what the appropriate decision should be? Body tension, muscle pain, and certain headaches are good indicators that an action does not feel right and probably should be abandoned.

Future Scenarios

With all the strategies for problems, it helps if you add a projected future scenario to your steps. This is a method of attempting to predict the consequences of applying a problem solution. Use the opinions of experts, your experience, and facts in print to project what is likely to happen if you choose this or that solution. Try it out at your caregiver support group. This prediction step will reduce the effects of *the law of unintended consequences* surprising you. These are undesirable consequences that you did not foresee but could have with a little futuristic imagination. For example, say you set an appointment with your attorney to get advice on a controversial medical procedure. At the time, it looked like the sensible and prudent thing to do, but there was a storm of protest from your receiver and family. They were upset that you arranged for medical consultation without consulting them—a consequence you did not foresee at the time.

Application Exercise

Choose a problem on which you have been working for several weeks but for which the solution is still elusive. However, start with the logical mode. How is it working? Then free your intuition and imagination to work for you. Apply the intuitive mode; then compare the two strategies.
Try multiple strategies with simple problems. Examples are: how to rearrange your sewing room, get more exercise, get the car fixed, get your hair cut, and shop for groceries in the same trip with a fixed amount of respite

time. Try them also with more complex issues such as whether to quit your job, move your residence, involve your family more in caregiving, or extract more time for your self-care.

Changing Unwanted Behavior

During the course of solving your caregiving problems you may have discovered self-defeating behaviors that you would like to change. One suggestion is to acquire more control over your variable moods that interfere with your life satisfaction and reduce your caregiving effectiveness. It is helpful to know that there is a procedure for changing unwanted behaviors and acquiring new behaviors, but they are difficult to apply in a self-care situation. Such procedures are beyond the scope of this book, but you might want to consult with a professional counselor who is skilled in assisting you to change your self-defeating problem behavior. How to find such a counselor is discussed later in chapter 9.

Communication Effectiveness

The basic rule in business—*Communicate, Communicate, Communicate*—applies to caregiving also. Your daily tasks will be much easier and more satisfying if you communicate well with your care receiver. People skills help to resolve conflict, clarify communication, provide support, and encourage constructive behaviors.

Communication Problems

Joan has a communication problem. She has been caring for her disabled husband for ten years. He has been bedridden most of the time for five years. During the last five years he has been irritable, argumentative, and critical of almost everything Joan did. She responded with irritation and criticism in her voice, too, so tempers flared and both were in an uproar much of the time. Joan says, "He doesn't hear what I say and he criticizes me for almost everything I say or do. Our meaningful communication is almost nil. Lately I talk with him as little as possible." Her husband, **Paul**, says the same thing about Joan. "She doesn't understand me and the pain I am going through. I can't talk with her because she doesn't hear me."

Improving Communication

Obviously, both Joan and Paul need listening skills. While your communication problems may not be as severe as Joan's and Paul's, nevertheless, you probably could profit from better listening skills. Even expert communicators who teach these skills continually need to practice their own listening skills.

Communication can be improved if we caregivers ask ourselves what **care receivers** think they need, not what we **caregivers** think they need. Even if the care receiver requests help, be wary, because helping is tricky territory. You may give what the receiver wants with the best of motives, but he or she may interpret your help as meddling or incompetence.

What is the antidote to misunderstanding your helping motives? Observe the receiver's responses carefully to determine the effect of your help. Your receiver may develop feelings of dependency, helplessness, or inferiority. For example, your receiver may think, *Getting this help makes me feel that I can't take care of myself, I don't like leaning on someone else.* Over time, such feelings could turn to resentment and guilt for accepting your help. Furthermore, it is easy to sound patronizing. Maggie Kuhn—a renowned advocate for elders—asserted that we treat older people like wrinkled babies.[3]

Communication can be clearer when the issues of how much responsibility I can, or should, take for the person is settled. Responsibility depends on the conditions, of course, but caregiver values primarily determine the answer. These answers vary from *I am my brother's keeper*, to, *Others are totally responsible for meeting their own needs*. The realities of caregiving are such that you probably choose to work in that middle range of divided personal responsibility.

You are aware also how your own needs for attention, power, affirmation, and deference could affect the welfare of the care receiver. Communication under these conditions is likely to be one way—from you to the care receiver. The ethical and understanding caregiver would not satisfy his or her own needs at the receiver's expense.

Effective communicators attempt to understand the other person. This understanding is a deep longing in people. Understanding people means attempting to look at the world through their eyes. This process is known as *empathy*—feeling into the position of the other person. Your care recipient appreciates this effort very much, because you are sincerely trying to understand his or her point of view. Joan and Paul, in the preceding case example, could have avoided the turmoil of their understanding if they had applied this simple principle of empathy. The important news here is that when patients feel understood they very likely will reward you with reciprocal understanding and appreciation.

Skillful Listening

Hearing total messages. To be understood means to be heard. Listening skill involves hearing and actively responding to the other person's total message. To comprehend the whole message, you not only listen to his or her words but also observe nonverbal body language and note feelings. Obviously, you are silent while the other person talks.

Listening for intent. You listen carefully and empathically to your receiver's words, intonation, and body language, but you are also actively trying to perceive what he or she is intending to say. People's words often hide intent. They may want to say, "I like you and intend to get to know you better," but some vague, confusing, and rambling talk comes out that maintains the distance. On the other hand, nonverbal signs, like sparkling eyes and outstretched hands, may communicate an enthusiastic desire to get closer to you. A psychologist once said, "Our bodies do not lie."

Your mental set. When listening to the other person, keep three useful silent questions in the foreground:

1. What is he or she trying to say to me? (What is her or his message or story?)
2. What is the person feeling right now?
3. What is her or his life space like now? (What pressures and constraints are in this person's present life?)

Attitudes

Helpful attitudes are an important part of your mental set. Here are some examples:

- Show *positive regard* for the person. This means a noncritical type of caring and nonpossessive love.
- Regard each person with *respect*. This attitude, supersedes biases and concerns about social status and ethnicity, race, origin, age, health, and economic circumstances.

- Respect each person's needs for *privacy*. This means establishing boundaries for yourself and for your recipient. Even close loved ones need their own defined personal space. Caregivers especially need boundaries to protect themselves from emotional overinvolvement.

Obstacles to listening. What keeps you from hearing the message? Usually it is self-preoccupation. We are so busy thinking about what we want to say next that we miss the message. If we do not like what we hear, such as unsolicited criticism, we do not hear. We also have a tendency to be inattentive if we think what the other person is saying is boring, irrelevant, or repetitive. Do any of these descriptions fit you? If so, how do you plan to improve your attention. Do you think you have an attention deficit disorder (ADD)? This is medical term for people who are distracted easily and do not give close attention.

Careful attending. Attending is one of the important aspects of listening. You show it by maintaining eye contact. This contact indicates intense interest and also is a source of information from the misty eyes or fluttering eyelids. This will not be a fixed stare if you are honestly interested in what the person is saying. Some cultures, such as Native American, do not place high value on direct eye contact when communicating. So, for all the skills listed in this chapter the cultural traditions of the person for whom you are caring must be considered.

Posture. Posture is a second consideration in attending behavior. Usually, when you show interest you lean toward the other person in a relaxed manner. If you sit rigidly or lean backward while talking or listening it may communicate disinterest. Even worse, hovering over people when they are flat in bed may reflect a domineering, patronizing, or authoritarian attitude. What is your posture communicating to your care receiver? Is it what you intend?

Gestures. What do you communicate with your body movements? Are your muscles tense and jerky or relaxed and smooth? What messages do you want to send with your body, and are they consistent with your words?

Verbal message. Beside content, voice tone, pitch, volume, rate, accent, and inflection say much. For example, your rapid and strident speech might communicate a message of criticism or insecurity. As you listen to your voice, what do you think you are communicating?

Your verbal responses relate to what the person has just said, so your recipient is assured you have been listening. As you try further to understand your recipient's message, you do not ask questions or change the topic. You stay right with the recipient awhile and avoid interruptions. A word or phrase based on the conversation helps to keep the communication going. Examples are: "I see what you mean"; "I can appreciate all that pain you are going through"; and, "Your idea seems to tie things together." This kind of verbal response also assures your care receiver that you are listening and trying to understand.

Why Does Simple Attending Behavior Work So Well?

Listeners like it because they get that rare experience of your total attention. It encourages them to continue the conversation and to assume responsibility for holding up their end of the communication.

You probably are aware that attending also has a powerful controlling effect. For example, intense eye contact has a riveting effect on the other person's attention. Thus, maintaining eye contact could help to control care receivers' dysfunctional behavior. (Do you remember the power of your teacher's intense gaze and frown?)

Guidelines for Attending

- Keep eye contact (in most cultures).
- Maintain a relaxed, yet alert, posture.
- Use natural, gentle gestures.
- Use verbal encouragers ("I see," "uh-huh," "go on," "great example").
- Find a mutually comfortable distance for every communication.

Restating Messages of Care Recipient

Paraphrasing is a method of restating your recipient's basic messages in similar, but fewer, words. This method tests your understanding of the meaning your recipient has communicated. Its principal value is reassurance to your hearer that you not only tried to understand but also actually heard the total message. Your recipient says to you, "Yes, that is exactly what I mean." An example of paraphrasing a message is: Care recipient—"I just don't get it. One minute that visiting chore woman tells me to do this, and then the next breath she tells me to do that [spoken with emphasis]." Caregiver—"You were really confused by her requests." Note that this illustration captures the essential message of *confusion* in a few words. The word *really* conveys the intensity of the confusion message, which was tinged with frustration. You look for a nonverbal cue (face, eyes, mouth, body) indicating that your paraphrase was accurate. Sometimes the receiver will follow your paraphrase with an additional verbal response, such as, "That's right."

Feelings are not always part of the basic message, but you must be on the alert to recognize and name the feeling. This is not easy, since feelings often are imbedded in long, rambling paragraphs. These feelings are reflected back to the care recipient in much briefer form and with a direct feeling label such as: "You are fearful of your impending operation." It is similar to paraphrasing verbal messages, except that the focus is on expressed or implied feelings. This is why it is usually a good idea to begin your response with: "You feel that . . ."

As in paraphrasing content, you will know when your reflection is accurate. The recipient will respond with something like, "Yah, that's it!" Even if your response is not very accurate, the other person will appreciate your effort to understand, then usually will give you the feeling that he or she intended.

How is this skill of recognizing and stating feelings acquired? Some caregivers have an intuitive sense of what the other person is feeling. Some caregivers, however, may have grown up in a family where feelings have been denied, repressed, or distorted. Others must practice becoming more aware of subtle feelings of hostility, fear, pain, disgust, sadness, or guilt, for example. Practice looking for cues such as misty eyes, twitching mouth, flushed face, and bouncing legs. Then attach feeling labels to these cues and try reflecting back your inferred feeling. You can say, for example, after looking at the pained expression, "Losing that job really hurt," or seeing the shaking legs, "That walk through the park this morning was very scary for you." Ask your receiver if your hunch was accurate.

When strong feelings, such as intense anger, are expressed it is so obvious that it is unnecessary to reflect them, unless for emphasis. An example would be, "You **really** hate his guts." Feeling reflections work best when the feelings are subtle and when the care receiver is hardly aware of them. Some additional example are: "You feel very sad on this anniversary day"; "You feel guilty so much of the time and so angry at him for setting you up"; and, "It hurts to be rejected by someone you love." Sometimes repeating the key feeling for emphasis helps, as in: "Her remark really cut me to the quick." You might respond with, "It really hurt."

Application. Practice paraphrasing the verbal and emotional messages of a friend or family member in the next few days to get into the habit. You can ask the following questions to decide whether or not your paraphrase was accurate. For example, "Was that what you were saying?"; "Was I on target?"; or, "Right on?"

Challenging Messages

In your attempts to listen and understand there may be times when you want to state your views very firmly, even if they are very different from the receiver's opinions. An example is when there is confusion about mealtimes. The caregiver may say, "I sense growing tension between us as we talk about this plan for mealtimes. I think we ought to talk about those feelings. Do you sense them, too?" Unless the person is mentally incapable of normal responses, this candor should reduce resistance enough to talk openly about feelings concerning mealtimes. At least the attempt to share feelings might reduce tensions to a more tolerable level and gain some compliance with mealtime rules

Send Clear Messages

You know from your experience how difficult it is at times to understand what the other person is saying. We are all guilty because sometimes we message senders deliberately want our message to be unclear. You might not want to get committed, so you give a vague, ambiguous response to a request, or you might want to evade confrontation on an issue so you give a conciliatory and noncommittal response. On a controversial issue you might not be sure what to say, so you give an ambivalent and garbled answer expressing both agreement and disagreement. The main point is that your caregiving tasks would be much easier if you concentrated on giving clear and direct messages.

Good communication starts with the simple principle of speaking directly to the person's face—never from behind or the side. It helps to speak calmly, in clear, short sentences, being careful not to sound condescending. This means thinking over briefly what you want to say, how you predict it will be received, and especially what you intend your message to be.

An important rule of direct clear communication is to give "I messages." This means beginning your statement with, "I think . . . ," "I want . . . , or "I think it would be a good idea if . . ." This rule establishes clearly the ownership of the message, instead of the usual, "We think . . . ," "They say . . . ," or, "Don't you think that . . .?" This little style change will increase the clarity and accuracy of your messages considerably. Thus, your caregiving tasks should be easier.

Questioning

The way questions are asked can either open or close off communication with your recipient. It is preferable to ask open questions that cannot be answered with "Yes" or "No." An example of a fairly open question would be, "How did your visit with your doctor go today?" (Not: "Did you get along OK with your doctor today?") Starting the question with "How" or "What" leads to elaboration and clarification. An example is: "How was your bus ride to the doctor today?" A more closed question would be: "What did he say that made you so angry?"

The direct and frank talk described here has some

risks. It may lead to a communication breakdown. On the other hand, it may lead to a communication breakthrough. The following guidelines may lead to a constructive dialogue:

- It is best when *the recipient requests* suggestions. If your recipient is not ready, there is risk of resistance or resentment. On the other hand, sometimes you just need to get things "off your chest." For example, to continue the earlier example of misunderstanding mealtimes, you may say to your recipient, "We have been talking about mealtimes, and I thought we were clear on that, but you have not come to eat when meals are served. The food gets cold and you complain to high heaven. I have become increasingly irritated at your refusal to come to meals on time. I think we need to talk more about this problem so we can reach some understanding. Do you agree?" (It is hoped that after this feedback the communication doors remain open. It is hoped also that you confront your care recipient in a tone that does not lead him or her to feel patronized or punished. One additional avenue to explore would be the patient's wishes about mealtime and your flexibility and willingness to compromise.)
- Give feedback or suggestions in the form of *opinions about the patient's behavior rather than judgments* about him or her as a person. (Note in the preceding example there were opinions given by the caregiver but no judgments. The patient was not labeled a "no-good, insensitive, uncooperative troublemaker.")
- Give ideas about *behavior that assume the recipient has the capacity to change*. (Assuming no severe dementia in the preceding example he or she apparently has the capacity to come to meals at the announced times.)

- Give suggestions in *small amounts* so that the care recipient is more likely to hear and not be overloaded. It would not be helpful to mention that you are irritated, not only with his or her lateness to meals and criticisms of the food, but also that he or she leaves dirty clothes all over the bedroom floor, spills face lotion in the bathroom, and does not flush the toilet. This litany may help get rid of some of your hostility, but recitation of your accumulated complaints would not change his or her behavior much and would increase his or her resistance.
- *Opinions should be given promptly* in regard to present behavior. It is not helpful to talk about unfinished business from last week.
- Ask your recipient for *reactions* to your ideas. What did he or she think of them? Were they helpful? Does he or she want to talk about them further?

Giving Advice—Does It Help?

The answer is that sometimes advice helps. Giving advice from personal experience or special knowledge is a common occurrence between people who know and trust one another, but it is important that you give your advice with caution. The reasons for caution in giving advice are that it is frequently wrong and the giver's authority often is used to mislead a gullible person. Advice also builds dependency on the giver of that advice. Giving advice based on opinion often is confused with giving factual information. The approach, "If I were you I would . . . ," is suspect since it often reflects the advice giver's needs, problems, and values rather than the receiver's needs.

In a trusting relationship, however, you can share your experience and knowledge confidently with your loved one. You probably know your receiver well enough so you can tell if your receiver is resilient enough to reject the advice if it appears not to be helpful.

If you are tempted to give information or advice, consider the following guiding questions: Are you perceived as a reliable expert in health care, psychological knowledge, child rearing, or caregiving experience, for example? Does this perception of your expertise by others build trust and confidence? How does it feel to be in the role of advice giver? How do you feel when people advise you? When has advice been helpful to you? Are you skeptical about the utility of giving advice? Do you offer your opinions with caution?

There is a place for suggestions that leave the decision about a course of action completely to the recipient. On the other hand, firmly offered advice is necessary in crisis situations where the recipient appears incapable of making decisions affecting his or her welfare. Examples are family readjustments after hospitalization or when your care recipient is going through a major health crisis.

So, You Can Make Your Life Easier

We trust you are convinced that with a variety of problem-solving methods at your fingertips and good communication with your care receiver your life will be easier. The skills presented in this chapter are to be applied in a context of love, acceptance, patience, and compassion. We understand completely that after months, or perhaps years, of caregiving frustrations your patience wears thin and "compassion fatigue" sets in. Under these stressful conditions, it is understandable that your communication and problem-solving skills decline. We hope this chapter helped you to put these skills back in focus so that your caregiving activities are not only easier but also more effective and rewarding.

In the next three chapters we will describe caregiving feelings of grief, depression, anger, anxiety, and guilt. We present effective guidelines for managing these feelings.

Notes

1. Robert Pirsig, *Zen and the Art of Motorcycle Maintenance* (New York: Morrow, 1974).
2. Eugene Gendlin, *Focusing* (New York: Everest House, 1978).
3. Maggie Kuhn, *Maggie Kuhn on Aging* (Philadelphia: Westminister, 1979).

Recommended Reading

Adams, J. *The Care and Feeding of Ideas: A Guide to Encouraging Creativity*. Reading, MA: Addison Wesley, 1986.

Alberti, Robert, and Emmons, Michael. *Your Perfect Right*, 6th ed. San Luis Obispo, CA: Impact, 1990. (How to become more assertive.)

Mahoney, Michael. *Self Change Strategies for Solving Personal Problems*. New York: Norton, 1979.

Marlatt, Gordon, and Gordon, Judith (eds.). *Relapse Prevention*. New York: Guilford, 1985.

Thoreson, Carl, and Mahoney, Michael. *Behavioral Self Control*. New York: Holt, 1974.

PART III
Facing Difficult Feelings

6
The Journey through Grief

Bereaved persons are like ducks—above the surface looking unruffled, but below paddling like crazy.

—Anonymous

As those of you on the care frontier know, caregivers experience many intense emotions. In this and the next two chapters we discuss ways of coping with the most common stressful feelings. They are grief, loneliness, sadness, guilt, fear, and anger. Even though your emotional life may be fairly stable at this time, someday you will confront these painful feelings. **Eva**'s care situation is a good example of how things can go wrong quickly. Eva, a caregiver in our survey, cared for her aging mother and her husband, who was retired for physical disability. All went well for two years. Eva was able to meet her caregiving responsibilities with satisfaction and efficiency. Then, in a short time, her mother's physical and mental health deteriorated to the point where she needed almost constant care. Eva's husband, while able to care for himself most of the time, also was making increasing care demands upon her. They could not afford outside help.

Eva resented the increased responsibility that spelled the loss of her freedom and increased isolation. She felt angry, guilty for feeling angry, and fear for the family's future. She was also aware that her increasing sadness was probably related to early grieving for her mother. Eva was annoyed at her own recurring arthritis and sleeping problems. She had long ago given up trying to satisfy her needs for intimacy. While she was receiving some help from her support group, she knew that she had to do something soon about her own emotional and physical problems.

Grieving

We humans all experience grief. It is a normal physical, mental, and emotional response to a significant loss. It is most visible in losses of relationships through death. It can also follow divorce, job loss, health decline, and loss of treasured possessions or beliefs. Grief is the painful feeling. Mourning is the process of healing that pain. It is a process of letting go of the painful past and taking hold of a hopeful future.

As we indicated in the chapter on coping, any sudden change in your life that requires a radically different response from the usual propels you into grief. Mourning over a severe loss is especially distressing because you have no pattern of experience from which to draw. There are no words to describe adequately the wrenching pain, searing sadness, agonizing guilt, intense self-reproach, convulsive sobs and aches, intense longing, inexplicable anger, frustrating helplessness, disconsolate despair, and fearful abandonment, to name a few of the feelings.

Because changes in your life are frequent, you probably have mild to intense grief most of the time. Do you remember the last time you lost or misplaced your car keys? Recall the distress, frustration, and helplessness—especially when you were in an awkward location.

Recall your last experience of grieving—the numbness, depressed mood, sleep and appetite difficulties, weakness, low energy, shortness of breath, irritability, anxiety, concentration difficulties, fear of your own impending death, and recurring images of the deceased. Your grief probably was experienced in your body as a deep ache, a craving, or an insatiable longing. Your chest, throat, and head felt tight. Your stomach cramped, and your muscles went limp.

Eighty-year-old **Josephine,** one of the caregivers in our survey, described her experience of caring for her husband, who had had a disabling stroke: "I was unprepared for the task. Longevity is a mixed blessing. Caring for my husband is like being with someone who has died. I am still grieving for my son who died thirty years ago. I moved to Alaska to be near my husband's family, but they don't appreciate me."

Josephine is depressed much of the time. Her self-pity led her into increasing isolation. She complains of concentration problems and sleep disturbances. She experiences very little pleasure in her daily life. She joined a church and goes to a support group regularly as her main strategies of coping with her grief and as her only respites from caregiving.

After the initial numbing shock and confusion of the loss subsides, a grieving person usually is flooded with emotion, as described by Josephine. When the person is able to let go of these feelings, there is usually a search for meaning in the grief. *Why* questions dominate attention. Examples are, *Why me?* and, *Why is God doing this to me?* Comforting insights often emerge. For example, grief can be understood, as C. S. Lewis said, as the price we pay for love. The more we love, the deeper the hurt when we lose that love.

Living with the Reality of Death

Since caretakers live continually with the prospect of death, they have constant reminders of their own mortality. Therefore, self-care includes acquiring a realistic and comfortable view of death and the process of mourning. The realization and acceptance of our common human destiny makes us kindred spirits and helps us to view death as a painful, but friendly, part of living. Sherwin Nuland, in *How We Die,* noted that when we are aware of our own impending death we can share spiritual companionship and final consummation of life with those we love.[1]

Pain and Loneliness Shared

One of our caregivers was willing to share her years of experience as a caregiver for her spouse. We asked what her feelings of loneliness were like. She replied, "As long as we could be together, in spite of the sadness of the disease, no sacrifice was too great. In fact, the busyness of the care tasks was an antidote for my feelings of loneliness and grief. For a while it was helpful to stem the isolation by inviting friends to dinner, but as he regressed, even this approach was unworkable."

What did she do then? "When the strains of caregiving became too great, I placed him in an adult family home. Now, robbed of my nurturing role, I was forced into deep isolation. I actually felt abandoned. The following year of separation became my grieving period. Meanwhile, I witnessed my loved one slowly dying in mind and body."

What helped her most during this sad time? "I realized that no one could take away my pain, but it was eased when I shared it. I think also that I faced my own mortality more forthrightly during this time. By drawing on my spiritual strength and discovering a saving kinship among my friends in my support group, I was able to pull myself out of the depths of my loneliness and grief."

Another example of facing the reality of death is the professor who kept a diary of his conversations with his dying wife. These entries later became the basis for a book on ethics. Writing and talking openly about death with him helped her to face this final transition with dignity and acceptance. His conversations about dying were interlaced with talk about meaningful living in the present and past.

Traveling through the Mourning Process

While there are no precise steps to this healing process, it takes a generally common course. Recent research indicates there are many patterns and pathways of mourning, including about 25 percent of mourners' experience of moderate grief that lasts less than a year.[2] For most mourners, however, there are initial feelings of shock and numbness, followed by a cascade of painful feelings, as described previously. Sadness dominates the middle phases of the mourning process and often moves into despair and depression. These sad low points can be a time of considerable healing—letting go of attachments to the lost person or object, letting go of all responsibilities for a while, and focusing on self-nourishment.

The mourning process typically starts a slow climb to more hope, renewal, and optimism and new goals and plans. The mourner comes to the realization that this painful experience will pass and that he or she will become a stronger person as a result.

If you are grieving now, knowledge about the mourning process can accelerate your acceptance of loss, increase your courage to face the pain, and facilitate the normal healing process. It becomes a time when you are forced to focus on key issues of life. We mention again Victor Frankl's death camp experience, when he found courage and meaning in his own suffering and in the suffering and death he saw around him. Another inspiring example is Isabel Allende, the South American novelist, who wrote *Paula,* a loving and soul-baring memoir, while her daughter lay in a coma for a year. In sharing her tragedy, Isabel rose above her despair and healed her psychic wounds.[3]

What Makes Mourning Difficult?

Unhealthy Family Attitudes

For some caregivers, mourning the death of a loved one is especially difficult due to low coping skills, negative family attitudes about death, and being "stuck" in the sad stage of the mourning process. Taboos and attitudes about death are changing, but many people are terrified by the thought of death. They use euphemisms such as *passing away, departure, demise, loss, final rest,* and *going home.*

Rosie, one of our interviewees, is hindered in her caring role by poor coping skills, low self-esteem, and a load of anger. She described a family background of unresolved grief and poor relationships. She claimed, "I'm not equipped to be a caregiver.... I feel trapped in this situation with my mother." The hopeful signs for Rosie are that she is aware of her inadequacies and desires to "become a stronger person."

Negative family attitudes toward special groups complicate the mourning process. For example, homosexual family members may not be accepted. Death of a mistress, divorce of a child, an abortion, or a family suicide could interfere with normal grief because the immediate family would regard these behaviors as unacceptably deviant.

Abuse of Alcohol or Other Drugs

The problem. Alcohol abuse and adverse interactions with medication are often difficult problems for caregivers as well as care receivers. Excessive alcohol consumption complicates the caregiver's mourning. Estimates vary on the extent of alcohol problems in older adults, but it ranges from 2 to 10 percent.[4] It is also estimated that late-life alcohol abuse is underdiagnosed and underestimated because older drinkers are less visible than younger abusers.

Alcohol consumption is an attempt to ease feelings of depression, but it only makes the feelings worse. Binge and chronic use of alcohol in older adults can have a more serious effect on their health than it does on younger adults.[5] For example, alcohol is absorbed more rapidly in older than in younger adults. The effects of excessive alcohol on relationships have been observed by all of us.

Management of alcohol. The problem for caregivers in managing their own consumption, as well as in their recipients, is to know how much is too much. Times of change, loss, and isolation can make a person vulnerable to alcohol abuse, even for the casual drinker or abstainer. As a caregiver, you can be especially vigilant during these times. If alcohol is a problem in your caregiving situation—either for you or for your patient—your task would be to keep consumption moderated, and excluded entirely when taking medications sensitive to alcohol.[6] It should be excluded also when experiencing sleep problems, restlessness, anxiety, irritability, or physical symptoms.

Treatment resources. If you or your patient is already abusing alcohol and needs treatment, there are several community treatment resources, including Alcoholics Anonymous (AA) chapters listed in every telephone book. It is estimated that only 15 percent of alcoholics over age sixty are receiving treatment, probably since special treatment programs specifically for older adults are rare.[7] So, your best resources are the self-help programs used by AA or the Hazelton Foundation Centers found in many large cities. The use of hard drugs is another matter that requires help of specialists listed in your resource directories.

Unfinished Business in Mourning

Another complication in mourning is the intrusion of unresolved emotional problems between family members and the care receiver. These residual emotional problems frequently surface as criticism or second-guessing the caregiver. This unfinished business needs to be *finished* as soon as possible through family discussion, even though it might be painful for everyone to do so. This means that the tension and resentments that may have been there for years finally can be resolved. In most cases, attention to unfinished business has a cleansing effect on the people who have harbored grudges, silent hurts, unspoken envy, and jealousy. It helps to reconcile the people who have been involved in the conflict so that they can continue improving their relationships.

Feelings of loneliness that have accumulated over months or years of caregiving make the mourning process more difficult. Words fail to describe the deep, inconsolable ache that is a part of the feelings of loneliness. One of our caregivers spoke eloquently of this empty feeling: "I live with it all day; the ache never goes away." Each caregiver must search for his or her own ways to assuage these empty feelings. Support groups and reaching out are obvious helps. Loneliness is not such a big problem when you are helping others. Acquiring a pet could help.

Forgotten Mourners

We caregivers must consider others who are affected by the dying of our care receiver. While we may be deeply involved as the primary caregiver, there are other obvious secondary caregivers who must be included, such as family members, pastors, physicians, and nurses. Less obvious are those who are not close to you and the patient, perhaps, but are concerned and mourning in their own ways—friends, neighbors, paper carriers, mail handlers, and members of community groups and social clubs. **Mary**, a widow we interviewed, found trust, kindness, and understanding from those who helped with financial details while she was grieving. While helping her with pension, banking, and Social Security details they also shared her grief and reassured her that she was handling her affairs well. They even apologized for intruding during this delicate time.

Anticipatory and Delayed Grieving

Caregivers often do much mourning long before the actual death of the spouse. **Catherine**'s experience illustrates this process of anticipatory mourning. She was caring for her ailing husband, who had suffered a series of debilitating strokes over a three-year period. The strokes precipitated many changes, including deterioration of his memory and personal recognition, declining control of voluntary movement, and loss of sexual function. His condition declined so dramatically that Catherine was aware that it would be only a short time before he would die. Her losses of companionship and intimacy, in addition to his losses of movement and mental functions, sent Catherine into profound anticipatory grief. She had all the predictable symptoms of depression, such as sadness, irritability, and physical disorders. She discussed her death wishes for her husband and described her feelings as being "on an emotional roller-coaster." When he died after three years of intensive personal care, Catherine experienced alternating feelings of relief and sadness over his death. In spite of these alternating feelings, she proceeded to plan her future with calmness and confidence.

Catherine apparently had completed most of her grieving over the preceding three years. If you find yourself in a situation comparable to hers, you should be alert to a possible condition called *delayed grief.* As the term implies, this is a kind of grief that appears weeks or months later—just when you think you are over the hurdles. It is a signal that the normal healing process is unfinished.

Having recurring feelings and grief symptoms later is normal also, but they are clues that you need to complete the mourning process of letting go of the past hurts and losses.

Handling Your Grief

Responding to the Impending Death of Your Care Receiver

In addition to our earlier suggestions for anticipatory mourning, the following guidelines and questions are likely to be helpful:

- Plan for a family gathering.
- Visualize immediate family members with the dying person in your care. Is the mood one of openness to words and feelings? What do you want them to say to one another? How do you see this gathering unfolding satisfactorily?
- Share your grief with your family and/or with your care receiver's family. Assure yourself and them that anticipatory mourning is a painful but normal process.
- What unfinished emotional business do you sense with your patient or others in the family with you? How do you visualize resolution, reconciliation, and closure taking place? Are there strong taboo subjects that would upset them if discussed? How would you handle these topics?
- Think about how you would fashion those last days for the person in your care so he or she could live fully in these final days. In your patient's present condition, what could be done to maximize quality of life? Without distracting from his or her need to discuss dying, how could you focus on how your care

receiver might also live these last days—smiling, crying with joy and sorrow, reminiscing with pleasure, or touching each other lovingly?

Cumulative Losses Intensify Mourning

Other losses contributing to the caregiver's anticipatory grief are loss of a job, reduced income, loss of companionship and intimacy, and, finally, loss of all meaningful communication. **Alice,** one of the caregivers in our survey, said, "It was the loss of all communication that was the most devastating."

Coping with Loss of Freedom

Losing freedom of movement and social stimulation is reported by caregivers in our survey to be devastating. It is fairly easy to adjust to temporary confinement imposed by caregiving, but extended periods result in loss of personal, social, and sexual identity. One of our caregivers reported that it was like being a prisoner. She spent much time trying to find "windows in her prison." She finally escaped her prison by carving out her own private space.

There is a positive side to this issue of lost freedom. Let us hear from some of our coping caregivers. **Doris** told us that when her ill husband slept or watched TV she went into the kitchen, shut the door, and listened to music, read, or just took time to think and doodle.

Deborah created a "window" in the prison of her small condo by making a private "nest." She took over her grown son's bedroom as her private quiet place. This spot became a larger window as she negotiated a change in relationship with her chair-bound husband. He would have to spend more time without her. She redecorated and refurnished the room, which became her private sanctuary.

Louise tells of her hobby of building and furnishing a dollhouse, which gave her some relief in fantasy when her life seemed to be spinning out of control. When **Alida**'s husband required a home health aide, she decided to take Saturdays off for movies, museums, shopping, and walks in the park. At first, her husband resented her absences, but she kept reminding him that she would be a better caregiver for taking break time away from home.

Mary carved space for herself by inviting her friends—who asked how they might help—to donate an hour so that she could escape her prison of constant caregiving for a short while.

Lucy, a long-term caregiver for her husband suffering from Parkinson's disease, felt her prison keenly. She liked to sew, but her husband, a love-to-fix-it type of man, irritated her by spreading his tools and broken parts of unfinished projects around the house and especially in her sewing area. He could not remember how to fix or reassemble the items, and he did not pick up after himself. Finding tools in the refrigerator was the last straw for Lucy. She discussed the problem with friends and provided a fix-it room where he could tinker and mess up all he wanted. She, in turn, declared her sewing room out of bounds to him.

Jeannette, a working single, brought her ninety-year-old parents with her from the South. Both were ambulatory; the father is in good mental shape, but her mother is paranoid and depressed and makes increasing demands on Jeannette. She became, in effect, a parent to her parents. She found her freedom in a nearby pea patch where she grows vegetables. She shares her produce with the local food bank. She is becoming increasingly involved in local politics—currently trying to protect the pea patch from encroachment by a golf course.

All these caregivers took assertive action on their own to escape their individual prisons. The self-help escape solutions were simple, but in our experience, many caregivers are reluctant to take these obvious steps to *make windows in their prisons*. If you feel as if you are in such a prison, we trust that the preceding examples will give you courage to plot your own escape. Use your support group for ideas and reassurance.

Resources for Grieving

Love and Sharing

The expression and receipt of love is a primary resource for comfort and healing. We continue our earlier caregiver interview on this theme: "Love was an important ingredient in your family. Please tell us your thoughts on this topic." "Love, for me, was not suddenly aborted with the death of my husband; rather, it became a wellspring from which I drew hope. Our relationship had been creative and interdependent, in which we complemented each other. That love has surfaced many times to fill that void of aloneness I described earlier. Writing was cathartic for me. Entries in my diary describing my experiences of caregiving and the death of my loved one helped to perpetuate that love."

"You shared many other activities that kept you close. What are they?" "Well, our music was another source of mutual pleasure, and offered emotional relief for both of us. I recall our nightly regimen at the piano, playing and singing together—no matter that the words were not always remembered, the glow in my loved one's eyes was prompted by the tune. Today, the song is over, but the melody lingers on! In my alone times now, I like to reexperience the inward calm while listening to relaxation tapes as we had done so often together.

"We shared poetry. One of our favorites was from Kahil Gibran's *The Prophet*. 'Our joy is your sorrow unmasked, and the selfsame well from which your laughter rises was oft times filled with your tears.' "[8]

"You had many pictorial collections of your times together." "Yes, my long-held interest in genealogy produced several volumes of family records. I used them daily as a diversion and source of pleasure for my loved one, who was fighting to retain his interest in life. As familiar faces were identified, it was like a renewed joyful discovery."

Special Support Groups

Support groups for grieving caregivers is another critically important resource. The power of such groups is the mutual sharing of grief and the resulting comfort and hope. The realization that members are not alone helps to assuage the devastating feelings of loneliness, isolation, and despair. **Lucinda** shared with us the idea that in listening to others' grief she no longer felt her grief experience to be as difficult. By comparing her experiences with others' she was able to ease her own burden of caregiving.

Healing Rituals

Rituals are helpful in achieving comfort, healing, and closure. A rite of closure, performed by our caregiver's family cited previously, was an important part of their healing and farewell. We trust that her sharing this intimate family experience will be of help to you.

"Our closing ritual was a comforting resource at the death of our loved one. It began in the hospital hospice unit. The family gathered at his bedside. We found healing together as we stroked our husband and father, wept together, and said our good-byes as we gave him permission to die. The nursing staff and our spiritual adviser, who were present afterward, gave us much strength to cope with our grief.

"Our closure rites continued as we composed our service of thanksgiving to be held in our local church. Our children celebrated through writing a personal synopsis of his life. Grieving time with family and friends, ministrations of clergy, and our community of faith eased the pain of separation and loneliness. The theme of friends and extended family at the reunion service was celebration of one who had contributed so much to life. I felt a great sense of closure after these events. In the following days, when I was left alone, the simple act of personally writing letters to acknowledge kindnesses and condolences was healing."

While rituals are helpful to many caregivers, early resolution of grief through rituals is not valuable for everyone. This point is illustrated in our interview with **Lily**, a spousal caretaker. Her only wish was "to have it over with as soon as possible." She exhibited no overt signs of grieving, and she desired no family rituals. It was apparent that postponement and denial of her grief led to an accumulation of unresolved and delayed grief. She is now trying to cope with this postponed grief in her support group.

Guidelines for Handling your Grief

- Increase your program of self-nourishment and self-attentiveness during these down times when you feel sad, alone, irritable, restless, and sorry for yourself.
- Be patient and kind to yourself. Stop criticizing and berating yourself for what you did or feel you should have done. Tell yourself that you did the best you could do at the time.

- Nourish the spiritual part of your being.
- Accept your grief feelings. Do not deny existence. Listen and respond to the messages from your body—the pain in your stomach, your heaving chest, and tense muscles, for examples. Speak to your body messages sympathetically and understandingly.
- Look for opportunities to smile through your sadness. Try to see optimism and humor in this trying situation. There is the example of the woman who visited her friend in the hospital after the friend had a double mastectomy. Expecting to encounter much grief over this significant loss, the first women was surprised at her friend's smiling comment, "Now all I have is edge." "What do you mean?" asked the visitor. "Well, I lost Cleave and now all I have left is edge!"[9]
- Write your thoughts and feelings in a diary, a letter to a friend, or a letter to the deceased or other family members.
- Join a grief support group.
- Feel free to hug, hold hands, cry, and/or throw things.
- Read how others have coped with their grief. A useful book is David Tredway's *Dead Reckoning: A Therapist Confronts His Own Grief*. It is a tender and heartwarming story of how he came to terms with his mother's depression and suicide in which he describes poignantly his own emotional emptiness, avoidance behavior, and quiet despair. It is a story of his own acceptance and healing—an inspiration for caregivers struggling with their own unresolved grief.[10]
- Recall all the positive and rewarding things that have happened to you recently. Ask yourself how you might strengthen them. Optimism can be learned and is a useful antidote for depression.[11]

- Conversely, be aware of the negative or punishing aspects of your caregiving tasks, and try to minimize or eliminate them.
- Plan to do something pleasurable, such as getting your hair worked on, eating your favorite food, taking a hot bath, getting a massage, or renting a funny video.
- Indulge in your most fulfilling hobbies and interests—favorite poetry, music, a trip to a gallery, walking in the woods, reading religious literature.
- Take good care of your health. Exercise is critical to controlling depressed feelings.
- Talk with trusted friends in your support network. Share your doubts, concerns, and frustrations with them.
- Take time to just do nothing. This is a time of healing, and you should not make strenuous plans such as trips, retreats, and college enrollment. Let time work in your favor to let go of the previous attachments first. Focus on nourishing yourself for a while—a good book, your favorite music, bridge with friends, and dining out, even alone if necessary. The African Kikuyu tribe has a custom of going off into the bush periodically "to let their souls catch up with their bodies." You, too, need this catch-up time.
- Be alert to mental images of what your life could be like in the near future. These are day and night dreams full of symbolism, mystery, and potentiality. How do they fit your goals, plans, and lifestyle fantasies? For example, as you struggle for new career goals, you suddenly are involved in an elaborate daydream about supervision of children. Perhaps, after your current primary care is finished you could apply your learnings to this new field of child care in a preschool or nursery environment.

- In the mourning process, there are special pressures, strange mixtures of feelings, and strong needs to forget everything and withdraw from the world. It is tempting to drown it all in alcohol, other drugs, fast driving, resumed smoking, eating binges, gambling forays, and other addictive pleasure-seeking and tension-relieving activities. Of course, you know in your more rational moments that these extreme activities are counterproductive and even suicidal. As the at-risk street kids are told, "Just don't do it."
- Be alert to suicidal feelings. They tend to occur in the middle phase of the mourning process, but they are a strong signal that a health professional should be consulted. Warnings are too risky to ignore. Similarly, take preventive steps with your care recipient. Older men statistically are vulnerable; 25 percent of suicides are committed by older Americans.[12]
- Keep daily tasks simple. A strong feeling at this time is that you do not want to do anything. All right, do the minimum to survive, but keep it simple so you do not compound your lack of motivation with accumulated work and household chores.

Gender Differences in Grieving

Do men grieve differently from women? The preponderance of opinion among specialists in grief work is that they do, but men in various cultures have different ways to grieve. Elliott Rosen, an experienced family counselor, concluded that men tend to withdraw from stressful expressions of grief. Rosen claims also that, given their social conditioning to be strong and controlled, men cannot be expected to weep openly in public. Boys were taught that men were expected to have "a stiff upper lip," meaning that they needed to act tough in the face of difficult emotions.

Yet, all the evidence indicates that men feel their pain just as intensely as women, who express their feelings more openly.[13] If you are a male caregiver, where do you stand on this issue? If you are the strong, silent type, do you wish to change your style of grieving, or is your present way of expressing your feelings satisfactory?

Child Grief

A great source of strain for caregivers with children is deciding how to explain death, disability, and grief to them, especially the younger ones. Children tend to take their cue from adults close to them. So, the extent to which you feel comfortable with death determines a large part of your child's reaction. As a caregiver, are you sufficiently informed and comfortable about discussing the topics of death and grief forthrightly and truthfully? Do you mythologize death, for example, by calling it sleep, a trip, sickness, passing on, or other euphemisms? There is much to be explained about terminal illness, funerals, and what happens to the remains. Most experts agree that children should be involved with the information, memories, and rituals.[14] Children should be assured that they are loved and can depend on care and security. Let them know they will feel sad for a while. Above all, assure them that their behavior, wishes, and/or feelings had nothing to do with the relative's death, if they should bring up the topic.

Multicultural Modes of Grieving

Since caregivers come from many cultural traditions, it is important to give a few illustrations of mourning customs to emphasize their diversity. You caregivers who come from cultures quite different from Western European societies will understand how some of our illustrations, suggestions, and guidelines might not be appropriate for you. Most mourning and funeral rituals in highly developed industrialized countries are quite homogenized. Therefore, little diversity exists except that kept alive in small ethnic groups.

Jewish

The significance of varied rituals is most apparent when we look at the ways other cultures mourn. In Jewish circles the *sitting shiva* custom is practiced. This is a week of mourning and close ministrations to the bereaved. Family and friends surround the grieving persons with prayers and loving service, so that the family is relieved of all household duties. For an extended time after that first week the grieving family members are surrounded by consoling friends.

Native American

In some Native American traditions, immediate family members assume all care of the sick and dying. They prepare and serve the food for three days before burial. Death is considered a rite of passage for the soul. Rituals are a blend of Christian and traditional tribal customs. One year after death, a "give away" ceremonial is held to end the mourning. It is a feast for all in the community, and each brings food and household gifts. The children participate and receive goodies. Fires are lit to signify the return of the soul to the spirit world.

Asian

While customs range widely for this large area, there appears to be a general attitude in many Asian subcultures that speaking about death, to either the dying person or the family, is considered rudely intrusive. Many are fatalistic about death and undemonstrative in their grief. An exception to this generalization is the Tibetan custom of reading to the dying person from *The Tibetan Book of Living and Dying*. These readings are about the princely status of the person and are designed to make him or her feel uplifted and joyous.[15] A wake may be held in the family home the night before the funeral.

Mexican

By contrast with other groups, Mexicans celebrate death and follow a mixture of Christian and early pre-Christian rituals. According to the Mexican poet Octavo Paz, Mexicans chase after death, hug it, and sleep with it.[16] A fiesta spirit pervades their annual celebration of All Souls' Day, when the dead are remembered and honored. Figures of ghosts and skull masks decorate the foods and are carried in a processional march. Dancing and revelry abound, and bonfires welcome back the spirits of the dead. Masses and prayers for departed loved ones are held all day on November 2.

North American

Since the cultures and mourning customs are so diverse, it is difficult to identify one distinctive ritual characteristic. Those death rituals emerging from the predominantly Christian tradition are celebrated primarily in traditional funerals, memorial events to remember and celebrate the person's life are common. While there is a strong denial of death in American culture, this is changing to a more accepting and open approach.

Some Final Words

Grief is a caregiver's constant companion, because changes and losses are a part of everyday life. Mourning is such an individual experience, but we trust that our self-care suggestions will help you through with minimum pain and maximum self-awareness. Your self-care will also help to inoculate yourself against a more disabling form of sadness—depression. If you discover, however, that your sadness moves into depression, you will find the next chapter helpful.

Caregiving is extremely confining when your receiver is unable to care for him- or herself. Loss of freedom, hope, and confidence poses a great challenge, but it should be encouraging to know that there are hardy copers among you who find resolutions. You can be one of them.

Notes

1. Sherwin Nuland, *How We Die* (New York: Random House, 1995).
2. Mervin Thompson, *When Death Touches Your Life.* (Burnsville, MI: Prince of Peace, 1986).
3. Isabel Allende, *Paula* (New York: Harper/Collins, 1995).
4. Pat Samples, Diane Larsen, and Marvin Larsen, *Self Care for Caregivers: A Twelve-Step Approach* (Minneapolis, MI: Hazeldon, 1987).
5. Ibid.
6. Stanton Peele, *How Much Is Too Much?* (Englewood Cliffs, NJ: Prentice-Hall, 1981).
7. George Maddox, "Aging, Drinking, and Alcohol Abuse," *Generations,* Summer 1988, pp. 9–13.
8. Kahil Gibran, "The Prophet," reprinted in *Selected Poems* (New York: New Directions, 1987).

9. Jennifer James, "Jennifer James on Depression and Aging," *Prime Times,* December, 1988, p. 1.
10. David Treadway, *Dead Reckoning: A Theorist Confronts His Own Grief* (New York: Basic, 1996).
11. Martin Seligman, "Optimism Can Be a Vaccination," *Monitor,* October 1996, p. 33.
12. Health Advisory Services, AARP, *A National Survey of Caregivers* (Washington, DC: American Association of Retired Persons, 1988).
13. Elliott Rosen, "Mourning, Melancholia, and Machismo: Do Real Men Grieve?" *Grief Letter* 2, no. 3 (Summer, 1996): 1–2.
14. Judy Tatelbaum, *The Courage to Grieve* (New York: Harper and Row, 1980).
15. Sogyal Rinpoche, *The Tibetan Book of Living and Dying* (San Francisco: Harper, 1995).
16. Octavo Paz, *Selected Poems of Octavo Paz* (New York: New Directions, 1987).

Recommended Reading

Caine, Lynn. *Widow.* New York: William Morrow, 1974.

Fine, Reuben. *Troubled Men.* San Francisco: Jossey Bass, 1988.

Hooyman, Nancy, and Lustbader, Wendy. *Taking Care of Your Aging Parents.* New York: Free Press, 1993.

Lewinsohn, Ruth. *Survival Handbook for Widows.* Glenview, IL: Scott-Forseman, 1984.

Westberg, Granger. *Good Grief.* New York: Harper and Row, 1961.

7
Depression: A Problem for Caregivers

Blues can hit us all; but they don't have to stay.
—Dr. Dale E. Turner

What Is Depression?

Extreme sadness you experience in grief is a normal response to the severe loss. This sadness, even though painful, is relieved in a fairly short time. The length depends on the healing capacity of the person. You also are able to do daily tasks reasonably well again, even though mild sadness persists.

There is another kind of deep sadness, however, that affects caregivers. We call it depression. It is a very sad feeling not necessarily related to your loss. It does not seem to have a clearly identifiable cause. It comes crashing in on you when you feel that you just cannot take it any longer. Or it creeps up on you slowly until you suddenly become aware of mental and physical changes like those of intense grief or burnout. At first you find that you are sad and irritable, like that "grumpy old man" or "sad old woman" in your care. Then, progressively, your mind malfunctions, your body does not perform properly, and your energy crashes.

Larry's situation illustrates this caregiver problem of creeping depression. He has been caring for his invalid wife of forty years, who has dementia from repeated strokes. At first he took his caregiving tasks in stride and took much pride in his newly acquired skills in cooking and housekeeping. He had been an optimistic person, but he became increasingly sad. His energy level declined dramatically. He could hardly get out of bed some days. Larry felt increasingly impatient with his wife and inadequate as a caregiver. He complained that he was a failure and threw up his hands in frustration and anger. He was going to his doctor regularly for sundry aches and pains that could not be diagnosed. What had formerly been sources of pleasure—his music and care of indoor plants—now ceased to interest him. He withdrew more and more from outside contacts and felt more and more helpless and hopeless. He hired a home care worker three times a week to help, even though he could barely afford this minimal help.

Larry's situation is illustrative of the caregiver who begins his care tasks enthusiastically, then slowly declines into frustration, sadness, and exhaustion. Finally, he experiences a full-blown depression with all the disabling mental and physical signs that go with it.

Depression and Your Health

Depression sometimes follows or accompanies acute conditions such as stroke or heart attack or chronic illness such as arthritis. Prolonged depression can also make a person more vulnerable to physical disease, partly because of its bad effects on the immune system.[1]

Severe depressions are thought by some specialists to have a biochemical basis in the brain.[2] This is why current treatment by mental health professionals usually includes medication along with counseling. Antidepressant drugs are improving continually and give fairly fast relief.

Depression is often confused with dementia. **Martha** thought her seventy-eight-year-old mother was suffering from dementia. She cried every day and was moody much of the time, forgetful, and disinterested in life. She stopped eating regularly and walked around in the middle of the night. Martha took her to a geriatric specialist who diagnosed her as having clinical depression and probably not senile dementia. A combination of medication, some counseling, and attendance at a widow support group slowly led to improved memory, mood, and energy level. Martha's caregiving burden was eased considerably.

This sketchy report of Martha's mother illustrates the probable *masking* of depression by complaints of her physical, mental, and behavioral conditions. It is difficult to perceive the depression in the mix of so many other signs and symptoms. Failing memory that older adults complain about is as likely to be a symptom of their depression as a memory defect from dementia.[3]

Mild Depressions and the "Blues"

Mild depressions are annoying and keep you chronically unhappy, but they allow you to function in your caregiving, parental, and career roles. Usually short-term counseling helps to reduce your feelings of distress. If it is any reassurance to you, having periodic mildly depressed feelings is a normal part of living, and it is short-lived. These feelings, known commonly as "the blues," overtake all of us at times. You just feel out-of-sorts for no apparent reason. It could be constant change or even a stimulating positive event like a marriage, vacation, or a new grandchild. Do you remember the uneasy, blue feelings you experienced on some vacations? Before grasping at psychological causes or dismissing sad feelings and low energy too quickly, however, we want to suggest that you seek consultation with a physician. Some of these low-energy complaints may have physical causes, such as fatigue, low blood sugar, or low-level viral infections. The baffling *chronic fatigue syndrome* lurks in the background as a possibility too.

Seasonal Effects

If your caregiving confines you indoors, or you live in a northern clime, you may be subject to *seasonal affect disorder* (SAD).[4] This is the depressive effect of sunlight deprivation for prolonged periods. In addition to gloominess, other effects are irritability, fatigue, concentration difficulties, and sleep problems. If you suspect that you are afflicted with SAD, obviously a little more sunlight, even artificial, helps. Keep lights on to brighten those gloomy days.

There is a depressive effect just from confinement indoors most of the time. We call it cabin fever in popular language. It is a mild form of depression and must be treated with the same guidelines for preventing other forms of depression.

Effects of Extended Caregiving

Prolonged caregiving can provoke mild to moderate depression. Caring for an ill person (especially if the person is severely depressed or demented) takes its toll on even the strongest caregivers. Even if you have survived burnout, as we described it earlier, there is a slow wearing down of energy and enthusiasm for the tasks. Take this condition as your warning sign that some temporary respite may be needed. But this condition is also a signal that a renewal effort might be indicated. It is like recharging the batteries in your car. Respite is a jump start, but the permanent solution is a slow recharge. You will find suggestions for renewal in our last chapter.

Depression in Older Adults

It is a common belief that depression among older people is more prevalent than among younger people. This is controversial, and the evidence is still sketchy. Our experience and readings lead us to conclude that depression is not more frequent in older adults. There are peaks for men after the changes associated with retirement kick in, but generally, older adults have developed successful coping methods for survival.[5]

Depressed older adults, especially men, are suicide risks. Their multiple losses, such as retirement, exaggerate depressive tendencies.[6] An implication for caregivers is that you look carefully at your own depressive behavior, as well as signs in your care receiver, for possible suicidal risks. Any suicide threats should be taken seriously, and referral to a mental health specialist would be mandatory. For your own health, it would be important to realize that if people are determined to take their own lives, it is difficult, short of constant supervision, to stop them. To avoid anxiety and guilt about this risk, assure yourself that you are taking all reasonable and prudent precautions.

Inoculating Yourself against Depression

What do you do when the person receiving your care is depressed and you are determined to insulate yourself against his or her depression?

- Insulate yourself as much as possible from your patient's depression by **being objective** about his or her condition. Do not let yourself react emotionally to the care receiver's emotionality. Use mental statements, as described in chapter 2 on self-talk, and stress inoculation. For example, give yourself repeated messages such as, *I will not allow myself to become upset about this situation; I will not respond with sympathy to his [or her] depressed feelings and pleadings, since this is exactly the attention he [or she] wants;* and *I will not reward that behavior with attention, which is likely to continue his [or her] depression.* Focus on suggestions for what he or she can do to feel better—"Let's go for a walk," or, "Let's play a game of checkers." Remember, you will need to use persuasion, since depressed people often do not want to do anything. When they are walking or playing, for example, they will find it hard to be so depressed, and they will not talk about their depression as much. You will have inoculated yourself, too. If you look at the patient's behavior from his or her perspective, you need not be so annoyed or depressed about it.

- It is important to remember, in caring for older people, that they were brought up with values and perspectives different from yours. Some traits of older persons probably do not make much sense if you are a young or middle-aged caregiver. Jennifer James cites several of these traits that make caregiving relationships difficult. For example, caregivers might label the patient's attitude as rigid or inflexible when he or she says, "I don't have to change my thinking at my age." Other annoying patient traits are fussiness, distrust, and anxiousness. After all, these traits are understandable, since older adults went through a severe depression and two devastating world wars. Other traits are *dependence* and *goodness*. There was a feeling "back when" that if one was good, someone

would take care of him or her. The trait of criticalness, which is expressed as, "I'm saying this to you for your own good," sounds patronizing, but it can be understood as a person's effort to be helpful.[7]
- Seek an accurate diagnosis and treatment plan by a specialist, as described previously, so you have a better perspective on how to manage your patient's depression.
- Carry out treatment directives from the gerontological health care specialist in regard to medications, environmental alterations, and psychological treatments.
- Follow the rules of good mental and physical health as a key inoculation strategy.
- Reexamine the self-care guidelines in the preceding chapter for managing grief. They apply to depression also.
- If the steps listed here do not inoculate you and you feel yourself becoming increasingly despondent, you should consider getting help for yourself.

Hope, Hopelessness, and Despair

Feelings of Hopelessness

Some of the insidious expressions we hear from caregivers who are experiencing even moderate depressions are, "It's hopeless," "I can't go on," "What's the use?," "I don't know where to turn next," "I'm a failure," and "I'm out of control." We label these expressions insidious or risky, because they churn and burn inside you until you reach the point of deep despair. They could be life-threatening also, because despair points to the suicide risk cited earlier.

What Is Hope?

Hope is clearly related to meaning of life. If you see your life as meaningful, then hopelessness is easier to manage. **Beth's** assertive self-care provided meaning and hope in her life. Beth's husband has Alzheimer's and Parkinson's diseases. Her three years of caregiving have been marked by his angry outbursts, uncouth habits, and irrational thoughts. Through the strain of it all, Beth's pithy philosophy has been to "go with the flow." She determined to laugh amid the tears, forego unnecessary housework without guilt, and make her own escapes. She solves crossword puzzles beside her husband at night and obtained a cat for companionship. Beth was able to think hopefully about her stressful caregiving tasks by saying often to herself, "This, too, will pass." By making her present stressful condition tolerable, Beth discovered that her life could have purpose and meaning. She believed that her life would continue to have meaning in the future. This is hope.

Hope is often confused with wishes. When asked, "What are you hoping for?" the person may say, "I hope I can get rid of this pain," or, "I hope the stock market will improve." Hope makes stressful conditions tolerable, yet it would be foolhardy to rely on false hopes that could lead you to disillusionment and deeper despair. An example would be a health condition that is terminal. So, hope needs to have some basis in reality.

Mary Lou, one of our interviewees, cared for her husband, who had dementia, for over five years. She shared her philosophy of hope for caregivers that she believed was based on reality. She was confident that her stressful emotional experiences could be managed without despair. She set three expectations for herself.

1. "Each morning I tell myself that I am responsible only for that day, and I pray to God for the wisdom, patience, and strength to do the best I can."

2. "Each day I try to find purpose, and even joy, in my caregiving; thus, I discover meaning for my life. This belief gives me hope that what seems hopeless can be changed."
3. "I give what I can to everybody, while not expecting anyone else to take responsibility for my life. My hope was sustained by the realization that my expectations were, to a large extent, fulfilled."

Mary Lou's experience illustrates that there is a place for hope in countering feelings of despair, but the problem is describing the desired outcome clearly enough to be a useful self-help idea. Hope is an expectation that the basis of the hopeless feelings can be changed. Hope is a feeling of assumed certainty that the difficult situation will get better and that despair can be avoided. This hope is maintained because the desired outcome is vitally important for the person. The hopeful person acts with confidence that events will turn out well. Therefore, hope is a firm, rational belief, as well as an emotional experience.

Guidelines for Building Hope

Rebuilding hope requires at least four courses of action:

1. Express your feelings to a trusted friend, care professional, or support group.
2. Apply thought-changing methods described below to remove the irrational hopes.
3. Mobilize your personal resources in the present. Draw on your relevant religious training and spiritual resources.
4. Act.

Move away from feelings of helplessness and hopelessness by acting confidently with hopes, ideas, and plans. Have faith in your future. Hopelessness, in a sense, is being stuck in a rut of confined thinking and immobilization. Reaffirm your ability to establish hope by reaffirming your personal coping strengths.

In the early stages of hopeless feelings, use the thought-stopping method described in chapter 2. Your goal here is to keep your hopeless feelings from escalating by telling yourself that you can stop those feelings.

Use the thought-restructuring methods described in chapter 2. Examine your feelings of hopelessness, failure, inadequacy, futility, and lack of control in light of these rules. You might ask the help of a trusted friend or a member of your support group to help you apply these thought-changing rules. While the rules are simple, it takes a high level of motivation and discipline to apply them to drastically distorted thoughts, such as hopelessness.

Perceive the meaning in your caregiving tasks. Recall examples mentioned earlier of caregivers who perceived their care as a calling, a labor of love, a service ministry. Reading stories of how others achieved meaning in their lives could help. Examples are Tolstoy's novel *The Death of Ivan Ilyich* and the Japanese film *Ikira*. Tolstoy describes a man dying of cancer. He was tormented until he realized that his life was extremely self-centered. This insight enabled him to change and to be reconciled with his family. He died in peace.

The film *Ikira* is about a man also with cancer who spent his life as a minor bureaucrat shuffling papers in a meaningless job. He realized that he had limited time remaining, so he spent his last days building a children's playground on an unused city lot. Thus, at last he found meaning and hope in his final days.

If your caregiving tasks do not consume your time fully, there are many opportunities in the broader community for meaningful work—paid and unpaid. Some examples are tutoring adults and children, working on political and social action committees or community improvement task forces, and service work with St. Vincent De Paul, the Salvation Army, or the American Red Cross. All of these lead to increased good feelings about yourself and counteract feelings of hopelessness, meaninglessness, and pessimism about your life.

The search for meaning in your life will lead to a deeper appreciation of the will to live. This is a life-sustaining force that, again, defies description because of inadequacies in our language. This will to live accounts for increased energy and many of the so-called miracle cures in medicine. It is a key element in maintaining and regaining hope and optimism.

Helplessness and Control

Some features of depression cannot be observed and are not perceived by the person suffering the depression. Such a feature is hopelessness. When pressures of caregiving seem to overwhelm you, the reaction often is to give up. This is a retreat into helplessness. Self-messages such as, *I can't do it anymore, I don't have the strength to go on,* and *I just want to curl up in a little ball and go to sleep* are examples that dominate your thinking.

Feelings of helplessness would be understandable when caring for a terminally ill person. In this situation it may be impossible to influence the course of events. So, you would soon come to terms with your core limitations and accept your helpless feelings. Again, telling yourself that you are doing the best you can under the difficult circumstances is good self-care.

Looking at helplessness another way, it is losing control. When we discussed coping skills in chapter 2, perceived control over your life was listed as a key coping attitude. If you discover that feelings of helplessness are part of your depressive picture, the way out is to replace them with feelings of strength, competence, and confidence. You can tell yourself that you are indeed in control of your life and start acting like a person in control rather than acting helpless and incompetent.

The thought-restructuring methods are helpful, but extensive reaffirmations are essential also. You tell yourself that you can go on, that you can tap your reserves of strength and that you are in control of your life.

A Look Back

Looking at this long litany of issues concerning sadness, hopelessness, and helplessness might in itself be depressing. The positive side of all this is that your efforts to lift yourself up by your own bootstraps are rewarding. Mild depressive episodes can also be viewed as a warning sign that all is not right in your life. Take time for a close look at your life during what little free time you may have. Welcome the solitude as an opportunity to get in touch with yourself, to meditate, to pray, to read, or to do whatever is renewing to your spirit. Be assured that your sad feelings likely will subside regardless of what you may or may not do.

A basic message of this chapter was that depression sneaks up when you least expect it, although in times of loss it is a predictable and normal reaction. Severe and prolonged depressions are work for professionals, but the self-care suggestions we have offered can ease the pain of common blues. While some mild depressions become chronic afflictions because of the grim circumstances of some caregivers' lives, be assured that much of the sadness will disappear as mysteriously as it appeared.

In the next chapter you will find helpful suggestions for coping with other troublesome feelings affecting caregivers. These are anger, guilt, and anxiety.

Notes

1. Peter Lewinsohn, Ricardo Munoz, Mary Ann Youngren, and Antoinette M. Zeiss. *Control Your Depression* (New York: Spectrum, 1978).
2. Molly Mettler and Donald Kemper, *Healthwise for Life: A Self-Care Manual for Older Adults* (Boise, ID: Healthwise, 1992).
3. E. Tunks and A. Bellissimo, *Behavioral Medicine: Concepts and Procedures* (New York: Pergamon, 1991).
4. James Luce, "It's Winter: Feeling a Little Down?" *Remedy,* January/February 1997, p. 10.
5. David Burns, *Feeling Good: The New Mood Therapy* (New York: William Morrow, 1980).
6. American Psychiatric Association, *Diagnostic and Statistical Manual of Mental Disorders,* 3d ed. (Washington, DC: American Psychiatric Association, 1980).
7. Jennifer James, "On Depression and Aging," *Prime Times* 8, no. 12, p. 1.

Recommended Reading

Ginsberg, Genevieve. *Widow: Rebuilding Your Life.* San Luis Obispo, CA: Impact, 1995.
Diets Robert. *Life after Loss: A Personal Guide Dealing with Death, Divorce, Job Change, and Relocation.* San Luis Obispo, CA: Impact, 1995.

8
The Triple Tyrannies: Anger, Guilt, and Anxiety

A soft answer turneth away wrath; but grievous words stir up anger.
—Proverbs 15:1

Coping with Your Frustration and Anger

Frustration and anger have been part of everyday existence since the beginning of humankind. Unfortunately, anger is the most difficult emotion of all to manage. It arouses massive hormonal responses in your body and dangerously affects health. Risks for strokes and heart attacks are increased by cumulative resentment.[1] This being so, it is obviously important to have satisfactory anger control and prevention skills, as indicated in Henry's situation.

Henry, a caregiver for his eighty-seven-year-old father, belatedly discovered the importance of anger control when he suffered a mild heart attack. Henry remembered that he had a long history of collecting resentments, but this time it was too much to bear. He had been persuaded by his two younger brothers to care for their widowed father in Henry's home. His brothers promised to help when and where they were needed. Henry's anger escalated when his brothers rarely visited or called. One of them reneged on his promise to send his share of support money. Henry's mounting anger was considered a key factor in his recent cardiac problems. He had some uncomplimentary labels for his brothers. Henry speaks for many caregivers who resent carrying a disproportionate and unfair part of the burden.

Anger, contrary to anxiety and fear, does not disappear quickly. It hangs in your being like smothering gas. Furthermore, anger accumulates in the form of resentment and grudges toward specific individuals or groups. Anger, like fear, was originally a survival aid. Its intensive form, rage, does not have a useful function in modern society. There is still a social need for "righteous anger," however, in the presence of injustice, prejudice, deceit, and betrayal. Anger must be directed toward constructive change, or it becomes a destructive force manifested in abuse, assault, or conflict.

It is often little things that wear us down as caregivers. **Judith,** one of the caregivers in our survey, said, "One day he was hungry for potato salad, and he told me, step by step, how to make it. When it was done he took two small spoonfuls. I was annoyed, and didn't think it was worth all that work." Anger escalates. Annoyance leads to frustration, then anger, and then rage.

Dementia care receivers are especially frustrating for caregivers. The San Francisco Family Survival Project studied intensely 248 primary caregivers. The findings, in general, were that in-home caregiving was hard on them and that they did not receive much help. Their dementia patients' average age was sixty-seven. Of this group, 48 percent wandered, 78 percent could not be left alone, 77 percent awakened the caregiver at night, and 84 percent were stubborn and combative. Half could not bathroom alone, and one-third needed help in eating. This group had been providing care for an average of five years at fifty-nine hours a week. One-fifth had not had a vacation in five years.[2] These brief data give some idea of the confinement and intensive care required of caregivers for dementia patients.

The employed caregivers fared much better with money to hire help and with a higher percentage of placement in nursing homes. One forty-seven-year-old care receiver's daughter expressed her feelings as follows: "One of the things I hate most is feeling like a prisoner of the illness. I do not work outside the home, and have no other local family. I hate the lost freedom because he clings so tightly in order to hang on to his only security—me."

Preventing Anger Responses

The best anger management strategy is prevention—catching it before it erupts. Recall when you were grossly misunderstood, berated for asserting your strong opinions, criticized severely, or the victim of injustice? You were probably very angry. What was it like for you? Do you tend to lose control in such situations? If so, the following guidelines will help to prevent your anger from erupting uncontrollably.

Controlling Your Anger

- *Listen to other points of view* before becoming aroused. In almost every issue there are differing positions. Do not hesitate, however, to offer your own position assertively and calmly. Argumentiveness almost always ends in polarization on the issue, with both parties becoming angry and often out of control.
- Keep in mind that *your care recipient may be trying to provoke you* with accusations, extreme statements, or attacks on your integrity. He or she is venting anger at the world, him- or herself, and perhaps you, too. Tell yourself that this is your patient's problem and that you are not going to fall into his or her trap

of making it your problem, too. Perhaps the illness is a contributor to his or her feistiness.
- *Respond calmly and understandingly.* Let your care receiver ventilate his or her anger. Try to see the world through his or her eyes or put yourself in his or her shoes. Ask yourself why your patient feels that way. Could he or she just be having a bad day? Again, seek an evaluation for possible dementia as a cause of the outbursts.
- In conflict situations fraught with anger, *be aware of any rigid attitudes* or inflexible judgments you may have made to inflame the situation. Remember, you are the one who is expected to remain in control.
- *Release your own growing resentment* in ways described in later discussion. Do not let your own feelings simmer without expressing them in some constructive form.
- *Avoid efforts to change a patient's ways* when it is clear that he or she is unwilling to do so. If you have been checking out nursing care facilities, for example, and your parent has no intention of moving, let it go for now and move on. Save your energy.

Here are some additional suggestions for anger management:

- *Tell yourself that this is indeed a maddening situation,* but that it is hardly worth expending your energy needlessly. Anger will subside after a while no matter what you do. If you act impulsively from anger, you might have agonizing regrets later for what you said or did. When someone behaves in a way to anger us, we have a natural impulse to punish the person. In the heat of rage we do and say things that harm us and the other person. Imagine for a

minute the regrets you might have if you followed your angry impulses.
- *Engage in physical activity* as one way to reduce the intensity of anger. For example, batting or kicking a ball or soft objects such as pillows and punching bags, allowing vigorous poundings to release angry feelings. **Iris** said, "I reach my wits' end sometimes. It helps to relieve my tension by pounding a pillow for a few minutes. At times I think it is my ever-complaining husband I am hitting."
- *Yelling and screaming* also reduce anger. But sometimes it increases the anger's intensity, so you should watch out for this tricky contradiction. Continue this physical action until exhausted or until emotional control and calmness are reestablished. Savor the feeling of relief and calmness. Consider leaving the situation and swallowing your pride, if all else fails. At least you control the situation.
- *Imagine that the person you are angry with is in front of you.* Talk to that imagined object of your anger with appropriately strong emotional language. Imagine his or her response and how you would explain your actions.

The Ill/Well Spouse

A frustrating predicament for spousal caregivers is the well spouse who lives long enough to become an ill spouse also. The newly ill spouse feels obligated to care for the other ill spouse, who may also move in and out of wellness. This frustrating situation is resolved only when the newly ill spouse can learn to be an ill spouse also and ask for help. Both spouses then discuss how they are going to handle their care mutually and how much outside assistance will be needed.

Abusive Behavior

It may shock you, but all caregivers are potential abusers. The cumulative anger from extensive and exhaustive caregiving can be so intense that the caregiver loses control. He or she then tends to abuse the helpless person indirectly by neglect or directly through verbal or physical assault.[3] All caregivers need to ask themselves if they are vulnerable. If the answer is yes, it is time to make that desperate call for help to a family or mental-health agency. In any case, it is a signal for mandatory respite.

This temptation for giving abusive responses to your patient is often a real human reaction to unreasonable behavior by the patient. Within their capability, it is essential for ill persons to learn to be more understanding and to behave with more civility toward their caregivers. A case worker could help interpret a spouse's hostile behavior to the caregiver if it is caused by physical conditions such as Alzheimer's disease. In this instance, the care recipient's behavior could be viewed as a consequence of the illness rather than as a personalized, voluntary act.

A calm, loving touch and a low, gentle voice may help control the dementia patient. Attempts to reason or confront usually will not work. Sudden movements should be avoided, as these patients are easily startled and provoked. This frustration situation is an indication that respite care is needed. Emotional distance in these situations is essential to self-control.

A caregiver who is running out of patience may decide to divorce an ill spouse, for example, as a way out of an intolerable situation. While this action may be taken in anger, it may be a calculated way to resolve a difficult financial problem. It may be easier to obtain financial aid for nursing care when the couple become legally separated.

A caretaker's abusive tendencies are just as likely to be taken out on parent- or child-care recipients as on spouses. This is a legal as well as a humane issue. Child and elder abuse is against the law in all states. In any case, abusive tendencies are a strong signal to get help before caretakers act out of uncontrolled anger.

Repeat Caregivers

Another situation producing resentment from our caregiver interviews was the spousal caregiver who remarried after losing a husband. **Carla** was the primary spousal caregiver for her first husband. After a short time she became the caregiver for the second ill husband. Unless the caregiver has a strong need to be needed, this caregiving reenactment becomes a disappointing and frustrating turn of events. Given women's greater longevity than men, this problem is likely to continue, and caregivers will feel anger toward their relatives for getting sick and sometimes for dying.

Forgiveness

Forgiving others for their wrongdoing toward you is no longer a strictly religious practice. It has become an important part of our secular culture. For example, the International Forgiveness Institute was started in 1997. The Promise Keepers, a men's movement flowering in 1997 also, witnessed thousands of men asking their families for forgiveness. Divorce support groups have incorporated forgiveness rituals as part of their healing work.

Anger and forgiveness are closely related. Recipients of angry outbursts have a strong tendency to fight back or hold grudges and hurt feelings. In addition, when someone does or says something to you that angers you, do you feel the need to get even? The need for retribution is strong, yet our ethical codes and civilized behavior call for squelching such vengeful attitudes. In most cases the person arousing your anger does not intend to hurt with his or her thoughtlessness, betrayals, abuse, humiliation, or unfaithfulness. Even if you discount the person's intent to hurt, you still need to be free of the tyranny of past hurts so you can release that energy for more productive work. You also must reduce your need to hurt others vengefully with sarcasm and ridicule, common means of venting anger. To seek revenge runs counter to forgiveness.

The act of forgiveness serves the interests of the forgiving person more than the forgiven other. Forgiveness offers a second chance to set relationships right. Forgiveness is a healing process essential to the health and well-being of the aggrieved person. If caregivers, for example, do not deal with their hurt and anger directly, these feelings have an insidious tendency to creep out later in self-destructive forms—drug and alcohol abuse, eating disorders, suicide, depression, and mysterious illnesses. Hurt feelings, as with overt anger, accumulate from childhood onward due to resented acts of parents, teachers, siblings, and institutions.

You are probably asking, *Why must I go through this additional pain to forgive someone I may resent for good reasons?* As we indicated previously, it is in our self-interest as caregivers to do so. For example, in a study of divorced mothers, those women who forgave their former husbands had less anxiety and depression. They were also judged to be better parents. Similar studies show lower blood pressure and higher self-esteem. The act of forgiveness does not absolve the other person of personal responsibility for what he or she said or did.

In addition, you could experience the greater inner peace, released energy, and joy that forgiveness provides. In the act of forgiving, you would take back the power to shape your own life. You would no longer remain slavishly tied to the control of others who have hurt you. Thus, forgiveness could be a freeing experience.

As a prelude to forgiveness, you could also tell yourself that the hurtful behavior reflected the care recipient's problems at the time. You could tell yourself also that other people cannot hurt you unless you let them do so. This is especially helpful thinking when caring for parents, children, and spouses who have hurt you in the past.

Guidelines for Offering Forgiveness

- *You must let the anger go* and stop "awfulizing." That means not hanging onto the hurt and anger to feel more miserable. You tell yourself, *I want to break this cycle, and I am ready to move on to other ways of thinking and feeling. I no longer have a need for these hurtful feelings*. Keep specific people in awareness as you give yourself permission to forgive.
- *It is unproductive to punish people who hurt you* in the past. Holding grudges and desires for revenge is destructive to inner peace, reconciliation, and positive self-regard. Vengeful thoughts retard the healing process for strained relationships.
- *Seek religious resources*. If these self-help suggestions for rethinking your hurts and letting them go are not strong enough to help you forgive, there are psychological methods that include fantasy and hypnosis. You imagine yourself telling the absent persons that you forgive them. Imagery, hypnosis, and fantasy work, however, are preferably done with a psychologist facilitator.
- *Share and rehearse your plans for forgiveness with your support group*. They can give you valuable feedback.

Canceling Guilt Trips

What Is Guilt?

Guilt is a big caregiver problem because you may think you have not done enough or what you have done is not right. Guilt is an emotion associated with some lapse or violation of morals or ethics. You feel guilt, for example, when you have not given your best care. Often guilt is felt when you experience intense anger toward someone you love.

Guilt is related closely to shame and shyness, because the basic emotions are similar. All three emotions have an eroding effect on self-esteem. **Genevieve,** a caregiver in our survey, expressed this feeling well. She thought that she was not giving her best care. She felt guilty about her neglect and indicated that this finding did not fit comfortably with her self-image of the adequate caregiver. She said, "It is as if I were living a lie. I knew I wasn't doing all I could, and I felt badly about that. Sometimes I hate myself, but what saves me is that I promise myself I will try to do a better job in caring for Aunt Marie. She seemed so appreciative for even the little things we do for her."

Strong Guilt

Guilt feelings follow from clear awareness of outright transgression of ethical or moral codes. Strong guilt feelings evoke a sense of unworthiness or feelings of remorse and self-reproach. With very strong guilt, the guilty person sometimes seeks punishment or censure to absolve the guilt. If shame is the dominant feeling, the result is likely to be strong feelings of inadequacy and severe withdrawal behavior.

Susanna, from our caregiver survey, illustrates the devastating effects of severe guilt. Susanna cared for her severely arthritic mother. At times the mother could not move at all. She urged Susanna to take some time off for herself, but she was afraid if she did so, her mother would need her. Finally, she relented and left the house to shop for four hours, fully expecting that her mother would care for her own essential needs in this short time. When she returned, she found her mother on the floor, where she had fallen trying to get to the bathroom. She was cold and whimpering. Susanna was shocked and immediately felt waves of guilt as she helped her mother into bed. Susanna felt bad the rest of the day and kept repeating to herself, "If I had only stayed home! Mother needed me and I wasn't there." Her self-reproach was severe.

Existential Guilt

Guilt for specific acts, such as in Susanna's situation, can be resolved with time and with rituals such as forgiveness, reconciliation, and absolution. Existential guilt, on the other hand, is a nagging sense that you are not living up to your potential. It is a vague, irrational feeling that your life is not right, but it is not related to specific acts of commission or omission. As a caregiver, it is important to be aware of this existential source of guilt as you question your caregiving actions. If, for example, you feel guilty some days for just being alive, you are likely to be experiencing existential guilt. For this type of guilt, counseling can help.

Social Value of Guilt

There is a social purpose, of course, for having guilty feelings. They serve as the social conscience to keep antisocial behavior in check. For some conscientious caregivers, however, their consciences work overtime. If this tight shoe fits, you might want to work on reducing the pain of your tyrannical conscience with its myriad "shoulds" and "should nots." Give yourself permission to let some of it go to reduce your fear and guilt. As a superconscientious caregiver, you may want to say to yourself that you do not care much about what "society" expects of you and that you are doing the best you can. Apply the principle of balance that we discussed in the earlier section on stress management. Keep some guilt as motivation, but let the rest go.

Guilt for Not Letting Go

A caregiver in our survey cited a source of guilt that seldom is recognized. **Joan** said, "My hardest task of all in caregiving was letting go of my loved one. I didn't realize until after his death that I would not let him die even though he wanted very much to do so. My good care and my energy kept him going even though he was suffering severely and too weak to enjoy anything. Even my doctor said he should have left us two years ago." She went on to describe her feelings of regret that she did not let him go sooner but hesitated to add to her predictable conflict and guilt if she had let him die sooner. She also needed to realize that she probably did not have as much control of his life as she thought. This experience raises an agonizing ethical question for caregivers. On the one hand, assuming you had the power, would you be prepared to let him or her die without guilt or remorse when it would appear that this was the time to go? On the other hand, are you serving the best interest of all persons involved if you keep her or him alive as long as humanly possible? Are you going to feel guilty if you neglect your care when you are morally committed to sustaining life as long as possible? If you slacked off on your care by request, would you consider this to be a special case of assisted suicide?

Certainly it would not be prudent to make such a decision alone. It would help to discuss this issue with a trusted physician, pastor, counselor, support group, or friend. It would be especially important to talk about your feelings on this issue after your care recipient dies. These discussions would be helpful especially in the event you had strong guilt feelings over your wishes for the care receiver's death.

Long-Term Care Guilt

Guilt feelings often are involved when deciding to put your convalescing or terminally ill care receiver in a nursing home. You ask, *Am I abandoning my charge by putting him there? Am I shirking my responsibility? What do I do about my feelings of guilt and shame? Was the move too early? Did I do the right thing? Did I have all the facts to make the decision? Was I really at the end of my rope?* Again, these questions and concerns should be discussed with a trusted friend or professional helper. When the decision about a nursing home for your charge has been made, live with it! It would not be productive to agonize over your decision or ruminate regretfully.

Guilt for Neglecting Family

There are so many sources of guilt in caregiving. One is foremost if you have an immediate family. The primary caregiver often feels guilty for neglecting husband and children, for example, while devoting disproportionate time to the patient. Feelings of guilt, shame, and remorse are too destructive to go unresolved. Let the guilt go and tell yourself that you are doing the best you can under the circumstances. View your time pressure as a problem to be solved.

Survivor Guilt

Caregivers, especially those close in age to the care recipient, report feeling guilty about being the survivor—the "lucky one." If it were an illness or accident that put the patient in your care, it is natural to wonder why you were spared and the other person suffered. This is especially difficult to understand if the patient was known as a good person who did not "deserve" what he or she got. If you try to add theological interpretations you get into even deeper water. Examples of this kind of thinking among guilt-ridden caregivers might be, *Is it God's will?; Why does this misfortune happen to such a good person, who has lived such an exemplary life?;* and *if I had only done such and such, I wouldn't be in this condition, would I?* These are unanswerable questions.

It seems to us that it would be more helpful to recast these questions into impersonal fatalistic explanations such as, *Being in the wrong place at the wrong time; making the best judgment I could at the time; There are aspects of my life that I cannot control and events that I do not choose but have to accept* and *This is a condition of aging.*

A Summary of Guidelines for Managing Guilt

- Decide if your guilt feelings are appropriate to your behavior. For example, ask yourself, *Did I neglect or jeopardize my care recipient's welfare? Is this guilty feeling a vague reaction to an unrelated situation?* Nonspecific guilt can be tyrannical and a demoralizing guilt trip that could persist for years.
- If you decide that you are responsible for the other person's hurt and you feel guilty about that, there is the route of forgiveness. If you belong to a religious

organization or church fellowship, the rituals of confession, absolution, forgiveness, and prayer may be helpful. If these steps do not heal the wound and you have strong feelings of remorse or self-reproach, it would be well to consult with a psychological counselor also.
- Give yourself permission to let the guilty feelings go. You must also convince yourself that this guilt statement must change from: *What a bad person I am to feel this way,* to, *This guilt trip is stupid and irrational. I do not need to feel this way. Today I will start thinking positively about myself and let those bad feelings go.*
- It is helpful to put your guilt feelings in writing. Start a journal. Pick a secure and private place to write. This is like a conversation with yourself, and it fits with the self-help theme of this book.
- Watch for tendencies to use alcohol to assuage guilt. If you are vulnerable to alcohol or other substance abuse, extraordinary vigilance is needed.

Banning Worry and Panic

Worry is a normal state of being, and underscores cautiousness and motivates careful planning. *Anxiety,* however, is a severe and unproductive form of worry. Worry often jeopardizes health and well-being. Anxiety is nonspecific, whereas *fear* has a specific emotional focus and is necessary for survival. A specific fear, toward snakes, for example, is a *phobia*. When fear reaches that intense point where it is disabling, it is known as *panic*. This is a sudden, short, often unpredictable fear accompanied by a sense of impending doom. Some common physical and emotional experiences during a panic attack are chest pains and pressure, heart palpitations and pain, difficulties swallowing, gastric distress, smothering sensations, trembling, sweating, dizziness, faintness, sense of dread, and fear of losing control. These panic symptoms usually are of short duration but are very distressing. They tend to recur unexpectedly.

Panic attacks consist of three or four of the preceding symptoms. They are doubly frightening because the heart flutters are often interpreted catastrophically as a full-blown heart attack, which, in turn, leads to more anxiety. Catastrophic thought leads to panic also. While panic attacks appear to run in families, the consensus of experts is that they are more the result of catastrophic thinking than genetic tendency. This type is known as "Henny Penny" thinking—expecting the worst. You may recall from the children's story that Henny was hit by an acorn and panicked, telling everyone that the sky was falling.

Henny also used another panic producer—overgeneralization. One acorn set off a generalized conclusion that the entire sky was descending upon her head. She had an irrational panic response to the event, too.

Panic responses add much misery to people's lives. Panic attacks usually follow a stressful event or a threat to security (such as impending surgery). Normal changes in middle and old age[4] contribute to panic attacks, so some are out of the person's control.

If you are prone to panic, your main strategy for reducing vulnerability is changing catastrophic thinking to positive expectations. In severe and recurring panic attacks, medications, combined with counseling from health care specialists, are most helpful to gain control of your panic states.[5]

The Worrying Caregiver

Caregivers are most likely to experience frequent generalized anxiety. This state is more persistent and less specific than panic. Anxiety may persist for several weeks as a distressing, but not disabling, condition. Anxiety is manifested by physical tension, jitters, trembling, vague aches, cold and clammy hands, dry mouth, tingling, elimination upsets, lump in the throat, flushing or pallor, being easily startled, high vigilance, and dread of bad things happening.

There are great differences among caregivers on what triggers an anxiety state. Worries about future finances, condition and safety of loved one, and your own health and sanity are a few illustrations. You could compile a long list of worries. For example, *Can I give the medications at the right time and in the right doses?* and, *What does my fluttering heartbeat mean?*

Caregivers have legitimate reasons for being worried, since so many of their life events are out of their control. A frequent lament from our caregiver interviews was, "I'm not sure I am up to the huge tasks and high expectations. I feel tense and overwhelmed."

Fearing the Course of Dementia

Besides the almost constant supervision of the care receiver with dementia, there is the fearful unpredictability of this condition. It has been described as the "never-ending funeral" or the "thirty-six-hour day." Not much is known about the causes and prognosis of severe dementia, so that the fearful caregiver understands little of what happened yesterday, struggles to manage today, and has little inkling of what will happen tomorrow. The unknown is scary; however, there is hope on the horizon. There is much research being done on dementia, and breakthroughs are bound to come.

Caregivers' Worries about Aging

Seeing a loved one deteriorating before your eyes is distressing. Not only do these observations about problems of aging give us cause to worry; they also remind us of our own aging. You ask, *Will I be in this condition of dependency and helplessness someday, too? Will there be someone to care for me?* **James**'s situation is an example. Following three divorces, James now feels trapped in the care of his eighty-four-year-old mother. Since she has Parkinson's disease and is subject to frequent falls, she cannot live alone. For the past fourteen months James has come home each noon to fix lunch for his mother. He says, "I'm just not cut out for this; I am a survival cook." Although in a strange and frustrating role, he likens himself to a disciplined samurai—one who does not give up. His greatest fear is that he might experience chronic and deteriorating health and get old and frail without having someone to care for him. He relieves his worries by target shooting and reading. His visits to a support group also help him to cope with his fears.

Jack Lemmon, the well-known character actor and comic, described his anxiety attacks at two crisis points in his life—when he became forty and again at sixty. His acting roles as older adults at these times precipitated his fears of aging and the realization that his life was slipping by. He controlled these attacks by making a decision. He would make a conscious effort not to worry about growing older. He decided that he would celebrate each new birthday with happiness and enthusiasm.[6]

Guidelines for Managing your Anxiety and Panic

- *List the things you are worried about now on the left side of a paper. On the right side and parallel to the worry, write down what you are doing or could be doing about this worry.* The mere act of writing the worries reduces much of the tension. Anxieties are not as fierce when you see them on paper. You can

attack the worrisome situations systematically or accept those that cannot be changed.
- *Do something physical:* take a walk, do exercises to TV tapes, or clean the yard or house. It is not only tension-reducing; it is a healthy distraction.
- *Join a support group* to talk about your worries with others having similar concerns. This sharing process is one of the best antidotes to poisonous worries.
- *Arrange a respite program* with a relative or other responsible person so you can take a trip, reserve a cruise, or arrange a short shopping excursion to escape the worry-producing scenes surrounding your caregiver role.
- *Apply the mental skills described in the anger-management section.* You can use the power of your thoughts to tell yourself that this worry is an exaggeration, irrational, or imaginary. Most worries are not real but figments of your imagination about what might be. Some worries are real fears, however, and you need to examine each one for its legitimacy. Then you systematically attack each one as a problem to solve. Consequently, you are in a better position to substitute positive and hopeful thoughts as alternatives for the catastrophic thinking and depressive mood of the worrier. Use Jack Lemmon's example to change your panic-producing thoughts to pleasant anticipation.
- *Take a deep breath and let it out slowly.* Repeat this routine until you feel the deep relaxation that comes with natural breathing. Furthermore, when you are concentrating on your breathing you cannot be worried, afraid, or panicky. Adding a relaxation routine will help you get your body and mind in a blissful state where there is no room for anxiety and panic.
- *Believe that you can control your fearful thoughts.* When you find yourself anxiously ruminating, tell

yourself firmly, *Stop it!* Say it aloud also. This thought-stopping technique works, but do not be misled by its simplicity. This is one definition of courage.
- *Learn to laugh frequently.* It is difficult to maintain a grim, fearful feeling when you are laughing. The worries melt into significance when you can laugh about them.
- *Develop trust in yourself and in outside spiritual resources* to reduce fear.
- Sometimes it helps to *follow Ralph Waldo Emerson's advice to do the thing you fear.*
- *Be an understanding helper* to some fearful person to allay your own fears.

Summary of Thoughts on the Triple Tyrannies

Anger is a serious caregiver problem because it is so difficult to express in the care situation. You can tell your patient what is making you angry and own your angry feelings. However, caregivers are basically constrained to sit on their angry feelings and suffer the consequences to health, relationships, and general well-being. The first challenge is to find ways to keep frustrations low and anger at controllable levels. The second challenge is to develop satisfactory outlets for release of your anger once it is aroused.

Guilt has its value to constrain undesirable actions, but our experience with caregivers leads us to believe that they have too much guilt and too many worries about doing the wrong things for the patient. The task in self-care is to transform that guilt into a sincere concern to do the best possible job of caregiving.

Anxiety is a two-edged sword. It cuts in a helpful way by providing motivation and energy to do the tasks well. It cuts in a harmful way by wanting to please everyone, avoiding creative risks, and adopting a tense approach to people and activities. The goal for caregiver self-management is to control destructive anxiety and turn it into a positive emotional force.

Notes

1. Walter Bortz II, *Dare to be 100* (New York: Simon and Schuster, 1996).
2. Family Survival Project, as reported in *Update* (newsletter of San Francisco Family Caregiver Alliance) 15, no. 1 (1991).
3. Kristy Ashelman, A study of divorced mothers, University of Wisconsin, as reported in the *Seattle Times,* December 21, 1997.
4. Arthur Peskind, "People Who Have Panic Disorder," *Treatment Centers Magazine,* January 1993.
5. Laura Foster, "Recognizing and Understanding Panic Disorder," *Counseling Today,* August 1996.
6. Jack Lemmon, "Decisions," *New Choices,* March 1989, pp. 16–17.

PART IV
Knowing Your Community Resources

9
Your External Resources

When the going gets tough, the tough get going.
—U.S. Marine Corps Slogan

Easing the Burden

A common caregiver lament is, "I have so many questions and so few answers."

In this chapter we suggest resources to answer your questions and reduce your frustrations. Many resources exist to give caregivers concrete help and peace of mind. The services listed in this chapter are only illustrative of the hundreds available in metropolitan centers.

Your problem may be how to access these services, since they are clustered in cities rather than in small towns and rural areas. In the Seattle area alone, for example, there are over twelve hundred services to older adults and their care managers.[1,2] If you live in a small community, check with your county agency on aging for suggestions and lists of services.

Even with the vast number of services, city caregivers tend not to take full advantage of available services. For example, the National Survey of Caregivers found that two-thirds of caregivers utilized only one service of a community or government agency. Reasons given for not using the services were: not knowing about them, not needing them, not being able to afford them, or too far away.[3]

The University of Washington Family Support Project provided family caregivers with information about services while teaching them basic case-management skills. As in the national study cited previously, they found that caregivers used very few services and that those utilized were for health care primarily. The caregivers in the project were an independent group that tended to view nonfamily help as welfare. In addition, families in the support project came for help only during a crisis, often too late to receive support from the project staff.[4]

While this independent, go-it-alone attitude is an admirable quality in many ways, it can make a caregiver vulnerable to at worst burnout or at least frustration. Admittedly, it is difficult to know when one must let go and allow others to help. Admitting a need for help erodes self-esteem and increases feelings of inadequacy for many folk. Imagined criticism from friends and neighbors about being incompetent or negligent is another deterrent to seeking help. A big reason for being hesitant to call in service people is a sense of pride: *Others cannot do the caring tasks nearly as well as I can.* We suspect, however, that the main reason for not using services more is that they are expensive. While it is true that home care services have been costly, an increasing number of free or inexpensive services have come on line. In California, for example, state-provided respite services have eased the burden of caregivers considerably.[5]

Care Managers

Care manager and *case manager* are terms that identify the professional caregiver. They will make a care plan and sometimes provide the care or access the needed services. They report to you—the primary care provider—regularly. They charge a fee because they are independent experts in caring for special kinds of disabled, frail, or ill persons. For some primary caregivers with good incomes but limited time and inclination to give the required care professional care is a satisfactory solution. Professional care managers are essential for long-distance caregiving to provide home nursing and health-care aides, as well as housekeeping and food preparation services.

Some service agencies have affiliated care managers who will, without fees, come into your home as a consultant and resource person. They will help make a care plan, suggest outside resources such as respite care, and arrange chore services. They will follow up on your care and be available for consultation on those big decisions such as transfer to a nursing home or hospitalization. They might even take the temporary care of your loved one under conditions such as the caregiver being disabled or suffering caregiver burnout.

Audrey's case illustrates the complex care situations that involve primary caregivers, secondary care assistants, and consultants. Audrey was responsible in her home for her eighty-five-year-old mother, disabled by diabetes, stroke, and dementia. Audrey, at forty-two was bedridden with paraplegia due to a childhood back injury, several recent falls, and severe osteoporosis. In addition, she is widowed with two children, both in wheelchairs most of the time, one from an accident and the other from a degenerative bone disease.

Audrey manages the personal affairs of the four family members from her bed. She is aided by a home nursing aide who is paid sporadically and gives most of her time free to this family "out of love and Christian duty," which is the way she described her motivation to stay with this family. Audrey has mortgaged her home to the maximum allowed and is in severe financial straits. The care consultant worked on providing a long-term solution to this family's financial plight, as well as finding short-term solutions such as respite care and accessing a network of long-term services to elders and children.

If you are thinking about hiring a home caregiver, Helen Susik's *Hiring Home Caregivers*[6] is an excellent resource for questions such as: How much does it cost? Where do you find a reliable care manager? Do you need contracts, background checks, and/or insurance? What kind of reporting or supervision is necessary? Even if you retain primary care responsibility, there are similar questions for the temporary respite caregiver when you take vacations, go to the hospital, or take care of family business. When you leave your home, there are many instructions that must be left regarding medications, managing the utilities, finances, emergency plans, and daily routines.

The following select list of organizations assists caregivers in their self-care efforts.

Community Services for Caregivers

Older Women's League (OWL)

Women have special problems of health maintenance, economic equality, and equity in the workplace. Since most caregivers are women without salary, this organization is one of the key support groups fighting for women's rights and equity. They have local chapters with volunteers available to help with the problems of caretakers and care receivers. One of their efforts is pension rights for older women. OWL estimates that 70 percent of the 4 million persons living in poverty in the United States are women and fewer than 25 percent of older women receive pension income. Another issue for caregivers is the large number of older women with no health insurance. OWL is working on this problem also.[7]

Crone (an Ancient Name for Old Women)

Support groups for helping caregivers cope with special patient problems abound, but they need a group like Crone. This group assists in their transition from caregiver to a new life of freedom from caregiving. While this transition sounds attractive, the prospect of change is frightening for many caregivers. Crone offers support through newsletters and programs. It is a global organization with numerous chapters. While Crone programs appeal to all older women, they are especially attractive to "retired" caregivers, since they emphasize fellowship, empowerment, and passion for life.

Gerontologists

These specialists on aging are usually in private practice, but they may be affiliated with universities or employed by research institutes. They assist caregivers with assessment of disability, give counseling on coping with children, and offer advice on managing work/family/caregiving conflicts. The problem is their high cost, although most have sliding fees. You will find them in your yellow pages. For lower-cost services, you might want to look at local mental health services, which often have staff specialists on problems of aging.

AIDS (Acquired Immune Deficiency Syndrome) Help Groups

Since a growing number of care recipients have AIDS or are HIV-infected patients, resources for the caregiver have grown. AIDS treatment organizations offer help with diagnosis, home care, hospital referral, and case management. An example is the Northwest AIDS Foundation.[8] You probably have comparable groups in your region.

Services for Disabled

Since many caregivers work with disabled people of all ages, resources are needed that are not for older adults only. An example is the ARC (Advocates for Rights of Citizens with Disabilities).[9] This local county resource provides support, education, and programs to assist caregivers and to promote independent living for people with developmental disabilities.

Services for the Ill and Dying

Many caregivers live with the fear of imminent death of their loved one. To ease this burden, a number of services are available, in addition to the counseling services of commercial cemeteries and funeral homes.

There are many agonizing decisions to be made about extension of life, specialized nursing care, hospital, assisted dying, funeral planning, autopsy, and organ donation, to name just a few. These are difficult decisions that you and your family make for the person in your care. There are medical, legal, religious, and humanitarian considerations. There are attorneys, for example, who specialize in state laws and pending legislation on assisted dying, wills, trusts, and advanced directives (instructions to physicians). There are also legal issues concerning durable powers of attorney (to authorize caregivers to make decisions for disabled patients). As you have discovered, your family physician is a partner in critical life/death decisions for the person in your care. If you are part of a religious community, your pastor is also a key participant.

Memorial Associations

Advanced planning for low-cost funerals can be made through memorial associations that are affiliated with local funeral directors. Most larger communities have these nonprofit associations, such as Peoples' Memorial Association.[10] These associations have procedures and consultations for planning a simple and inexpensive funeral or memorial service. They help with handling the body and meeting legal requirements, such as death certificates and media notifications. It would be a prudent idea to discuss with your loved one in your care and close relatives the issues and needs for planning raised previously. It may be difficult for you, but it is essential that your preferences and your patient's wishes are known to the entire family. This planning is part of your self-care package. It will help reduce potential stressors when death occurs. This plan should be well-known by all concerned and not tucked away obscurely in the will.

Right to Die

Since you may be caring for a terminally ill person, there are services to help with decisions in the last days of life. States are rapidly passing and improving their right-to-die statutes. An example of a nonprofit organization dedicated to helping with end-of-life issues is Washington's Compassion in Dying. There probably is a comparable group in your state. Its general purpose is to assure a humane and dignified death and to enhance the celebration of life. Specifically, such organizations provide information and counseling for families. They also offer emotional support to terminally ill patients who are trying to decide how and when their lives will end.

Hemlock Society

If end-of-life services meet your needs, inquire at your local medical association, county office on aging, or local Hemlock Society for information. Many communities have Hemlock Society chapters that offer information and counseling on planning for those last days of life. They assist in clarification of the profound values that the dying person must consider in a life/death decision and assist caregivers with suggestions for approaching your care recipient on such issues as living wills, powers of attorney, and advance directives.

Hospice

Hospice programs are available, usually through hospitals, to assist caregivers with services for the terminally ill. Their round-the-clock support and pain management, spiritual and grief counseling, pastoral care, and grief support groups are their main services. Families are the unit of care in hospice programs, whether in the home or the hospital. Hospice care usually begins about six months before the estimated time of death.

One of the unique features of hospice programs is that they emphasize life before death. These programs include ways to maintain quality of life until the end. So often when people receive the diagnosis of terminal illness they are treated as if they were already gone. In the worst scenarios, they are shunted aside and ignored. Hospice programs seek to avoid this indignity.

Visiting Nurse Services

In addition to work with the terminally ill, visiting nurse services come to the caregiver's home to offer counseling, health care, and advice on accessing community health services. Some health-maintenance organizations provide this service as part of their health insurance program. Check your policy for this provision.

Chore Services and Respite Care

Increasing numbers of community-based services are available for doing light household chores at low fees. Similarly, low-cost respite care by volunteers or paid workers is a recent development to ease the burden on caregivers. Just having a few hours a week for shopping, hair care, and medical/dental appointments is a major boost for the confined caregiver.

Elder Care Locator

This is a nation-wide American locator system. It provides community information and network referral for local services to elders. See notes for contact information.[11]

American Association for Retired Persons

This organization (AARP) has several resources for caregivers. The national group publishes helpful pamphlets on many topics related to care, such as how to adapt your home for a disabled person. They distribute a collection called the Caregiver's Resource Kit.[12] Local chapters have volunteers working on projects to assist caregivers with such decisions as long-term care and retirement.

Religious Resources

Values of Religious Affiliation

Organized religious groups offer helpful resources to deepen your spirituality. Caregivers who have retained affiliation with a religious community know the personal values of ritual, confession, absolution, reconciliation, and forgiveness. Rituals can lead to spiritual heights of celebration, reverence for the sacred, holiness, and transcendence. Most important, a religious organization offers the support of a caring community. Many churches provide pastoral service to visit shut-ins, arrange respite, and offer comfort to the bereaved. Thus, these institutional services are valuable resources for caregivers.

At a personal level, a religious environment offers opportunities to review, expand, and clarify your caregiving service. In addition, such a connection can help you confront your purpose for living and the meaning of life. With increasing involvement of religious groups in social issues and politics, there are additional opportunities to clarify your views on the relevance of your spiritual commitment to public policy and government. Where do you stand on public housing, welfare, Medicaid, and subsidized child care, for example?

Handling Negative Attitudes

Some caregivers are skeptical about the value of institutionalized religion because of negative or neutral experiences in younger years. Some are turned off by incessant appeals for money or time. If this description fits you, but you want to reestablish your ties with an organized religious group, you must first let go of those cumulative negative feelings and refocus your image of that group. So, as a current or prospective caregiver, you might want to examine your present attitudes about formal religion through counseling. Then make a considered judgment about how a religious commitment might or might not assist you in spending your caregiving years with more satisfaction. You can tell yourself, for example, that this situation exists for you—not the reverse. You can reexperience the previous meaningless rituals in such a way that they would have more personal meaning and be more energizing now. You can also tell yourself that the purpose of religious authority is "to build you up, not put you down." Recall our earlier discussion on changing thoughts and attitudes.

Whether your religious commitment is Christian, Jewish, Islamic, Buddhist, Bahai, or Native American naturalist, for example, you can look profitably at the comment of Jesus, who said, "I have come that you might have life, and have it more abundantly"—more spirit, energy, wholeness, belonging, purpose, and fulfillment. Other religious leaders have made similar life-affirming declarations.

Relationship to Physical Health

There is growing evidence that a strong religious faith, combined with rituals of prayer and meditation, contributes to physical healing and disease prevention.[13] The Care-Net study of the Carter Foundation found that caregivers with a strong religious faith were less likely to experience burnout than those without such a sustaining religious faith.[14]

Support Services for Caregivers

The value of giving and receiving support as a coping skill was described in chapter 2. This section represents community services that give direct emotional and informational support to caregivers.

Support Groups

Support groups are essential for caregiver survival. They provide information, emotional sustenance, encouragement, and personal growth. They are not psychotherapy groups, although the results usually are therapeutic. Members talk about their common concerns, information needs, and feelings about caregiving.

Groups are useful throughout the entire time of care, but especially those first weeks. **Lena**'s situation illustrates: "It was hard for me to realize the seriousness and enormousness of the task. When my mother was diagnosed with Alzheimer's disease, I was not surprised; rather, I was overwhelmed by the thought of giving her total care. A friend suggested I check into a support group. It was such a great help. They were kind and understanding, and gave me a lot of good suggestions that I hadn't thought of before about the illness and its legal and medical considerations. They also helped me with the decision about nursing homes. I was beginning to feel so guilty at just the thought of it."

The first few weeks are a critical adjustment time, as Lena's situation illustrates. If you are a caregiver now or anticipate such a role soon, it would help greatly to know that there are special groups able and willing to assist you through those difficult first weeks. You would realize that you are not alone, for example. Sometimes it takes time to comprehend that you have a serious problem. A support group can help you see that problem more clearly. They can suggest ways to approach issues, such as realizing that you have a "new child" at home, in terms of care requirements. Members of the group often are willing to serve on a telephone network so they are available around-the-clock. One early issue that comes up invariably, as it did for Lena, is the decision whether to continue care by yourself or consider a nursing home, with all the complications of money, separation, and guilt.

Problems with Support Groups

There **are** some problems connected with support groups. They are not for everyone, since most people are not comfortable sharing personal information in intimate groups. There are so many special focus groups that it takes some research to find the right one. There are, for example, dementia, stroke, cardiac, alcoholic, widow, divorce, parenting, and nonspecific women's and men's groups. It is essential to stay with the group long enough to feel comfortable and experience mutual trust. There is also the obligation to attend the group regularly.

Structure of Support Groups

Groups usually meet bimonthly, so the problem of finding respite care while you are attending might be a continuing concern. Your network of friends, family, church members, or community senior service organizations is useful here to provide the respite time to attend regular support group meetings. Some groups do not have a professional leader, called a *facilitator*. Therefore, leadership emerges from the group. Having a designated leader has some advantages in keeping the group on track and ensuring that all have a chance to participate.

The greatest problem for caregivers is finding time to squeeze in one more commitment, especially if you spend forty hours a week employed and another forty to sixty hours in caregiving. On the optimistic side, however, is that large businesses are developing programs for combining caregiving and employment. They include support networks and groups, along with flex time, day care, and respite services. They find this plan creates more-satisfied employees and helps productivity. If you do not have these opportunities at work, assert your leadership by proposing such a program to your employer.

Members of support groups develop friendships that sustain them long beyond the confining period of caregiving. Grief support when the person dies is an example of such continuity. If you are a male caregiver and do not feel comfortable in mixed-sex support groups, there are growing numbers of men's support groups emerging.

Support groups are organized by hospitals, mental-health clinics, associations, churches, and senior centers. They usually have no fees, but they ask for a commitment. You are asked to subscribe to some affirmations and guidelines, such as maintaining confidentiality, accepting other members without judgment, sharing time equitably, and being willing to share your concerns and feelings.

Eldercare Services by Corporations

A growing number of companies have established caregiving referral services for elders that are comparable to child-care services. IBM is an example in which higher productivity and morale resulted from such service.[15] If you are an employed caregiver, check with your employer about their support program.

Computer Internet

The Internet is a fast-growing source of information on caregiving. An example is the Web site established and maintained by the Family Caregiver Alliance of San Francisco. This site can be accessed through www.caregiver.org. It provides news on public policy legislation, a clearinghouse for facts, a resource center for advice, and linkage to other sites. In Appendix B you will find a list of Web sites useful to caregivers.

Networking

In addition to organized groups, communities are interlaced with informal networks of people who have common goals and needs. These are relatives and acquaintances acquired over the years with whom you still have some connection. Utilizing informal service networks systems and formal service systems is no problem for the caregiver who has lived in the same community for several years.[16] If you are a newcomer, it will take special effort to join or build such a network and to become familiar with community services.

Counseling

When the pressures accumulate and the prospects of burnout harm you, it may be time to seek counseling before a major crisis develops. Counseling enables you to solve your own problems in a safe and trusting atmosphere and to take charge of your own life. The counselor acts as guide, facilitator, and resource person.

The problems faced by **Irene,** a stressed-out caregiver, illustrate the eventual need for counseling. She was depressed and fatigued after five years of caring for her husband, who had had multiple strokes. Irene felt her situation was hopeless and all she could think about and wish for was his death. She was frustrated over the loss of their former loving relationship and intimacy.

Irene had become increasingly isolated, although she had occasional telephone visits with her daughter, Fay, who lived in a distant city. From telephone conversations and after a recent visit Fay became alarmed about her mother's deteriorating emotional condition and thought her mother should get counseling. Fay contacted the local mental health center to make an appointment with a geriatric counselor. Irene was reluctant and fearful at first about revealing facts from her personal life. Fay's persuasion and offer to pay the fees convinced her to try it. Fay arranged the respite care for Irene's invalid husband also. The counseling went quite well over the next few weeks. Irene grieved for her losses, aired her feelings, and was assured that she was not mentally ill. She started to exercise more, developed a more optimistic outlook on her life, and gained more objectivity about her husband's disability.

Styles of Counseling

There are different styles of counseling suited to different problems, so choice is difficult. If you decide to try counseling, recommendations of friends who have received counseling recently from a particular person are your best sources. You might ask for suggestions from one of your professional consultants, care manager, or a local professional association. Then give it a try, and if this is not the right person or style, try another. The personal fit needs to be right to develop a trusting relationship. The problem again is cost. Fees for private practice, even if they are in a managed-care program, are sixty dollars to ninety dollars and more per hour. Many counselors have sliding fees, and public mental health clinics offer services at lower cost than private practitioners.

Counselor Credentials

Deciding on the type of counselor complicates **your** choice, too. There are licensed professional mental health counselors who have at least a master's degree. Licensed psychologists have Ph.D. degrees and offer psychotherapeutic types of counseling as well as assistance with choices such as careers, lifestyle, addictions, and retirement. Licensed psychiatrists have M.D. degrees and offer psychotherapy services with medicinal treatment, if indicated. Clinical social workers usually have M.S.W. degrees and offer a wide range of counseling assistance to caregivers. They know community resources well, since this is part of their graduate training. Pastoral counselors, who often have extensive psychological training, offer counseling services also.

This is a sketchy picture of the counseling scene, so when that time comes to make this choice you can do more extensive research to find the best type of counselor for you. Keep in mind that counseling does not need to be long-term. You can commit yourself to short periods, such as a few weeks, for working on immediate problems. Brief therapy usually covers one to ten sessions. Thus, you could achieve sufficient stability to continue your caregiving responsibilities with confidence and satisfaction.

A Last Word on Resources

This list of external caregiver resources is only a sample of hundreds available. The moral of this study is to use the services for vital information and to lighten your burden. Get on the mailing list of your local area agency on aging to stay current about new services.

Notes

1. Robert Daniel, *Aging Well: The Older Adults' Resource Directory* (Seattle: Watermark, 1997).
2. Jean Quam, *Social Services for Older Gay Men and Lesbians* (Binghamton, NY: Haworth, 1996).
3. Opinion Research Corporation (for AARP). *A National Survey of Caregivers* (Washington, DC: American Association of Retired Persons, 1988).
4. Rhonda Montgomery, *Family Support Project* (final report) (Washington, DC: Administration on Aging, U.S. Department of Health and Human Services, 1985).
5. Family Survival Project, *Update* 10, No. 4 (Winter, 1992): 1.
6. Helen Susik, *Hiring Home Caregivers* (San Luis Obispo, CA: Impact, 1995).
7. Older Women's League. *Women and Pensions* (Washington, DC: Older Women's League, 1996).
8. Northwest AIDS Foundation, *Services for People with AIDS and HIV* (Seattle: Northwest AIDS Foundation, 1996).
9. ARC. *The ARC* (Seattle, WA: ARC, 1996).
10. People's Memorial Association, *Planning for Simpler Funerals* (Seattle, WA: People's Memorial Association, 1995); Van Tuyl (ed.), *What You Should Know about Death Services* (Seattle, WA: People's Memorial Association, 1991).

11. U.S. Department of Health and Human Services, Administration on Aging "Elder Care Locator: A Way to Find Community Assistance for Seniors," 1-800-677-1116, Mon.–Fri., 9:00 A.M. to 11:00 P.M. EST.
12. American Association of Retired Persons, Publication D 15267, Caregivers Resource Kit (a collection of useful pamphlets on caregiving resources) (Washington, DC: AARP, 1994).
13. Wayne Miller, *Legacy of the Heart* (New York: Bantam, 1995).
14. Jack Nottingham, "Care Net Study," reported in *Caregivers and Caregiving in West Central Georgia* (Americus, GA: Rosalynn Carter Institute, 1993).
15. *Mature Outlook Newsletter,* Fall 1996, p. 6.
16. Eugene Liwak, *Helping the Elderly: The Complementary Roles of Informal and Formal Systems* (New York: Guilford, 1990).

Recommended Reading

American Heart Association. *Stroke Connection.* (Dallas, TX: American Heart Association, n.d.) (A nationwide resource for stroke survivors; also produces newsletters *Stroke Connection,* for stroke patients, and *A Stroke of Luck,* for people with aphasia.)

Dippel, Raye, and Sutton, J. Thomas (eds.). *Caring for the Alzheimer Patient: A Practical Guide,* 3d ed. New York: Prometheus, 1996.

Family Caregiver Alliance. *Caregiver Fact Sheets Online.* Family Caregiver Alliance Web Site HTTP://www.caregiver.org.

Group Health Cooperative. *Consumer Guide to Advanced Directives.* Seattle, WA: Group Health Cooperative Advance Directives. Central Hospital, 1992. (How to plan living wills, durable powers of attorney, and advanced directives.)

Hutton, Thomas J. (ed.). *Caring for the Parkinson Patient.* New York: Prometheus, 1994.

Quinn, Terry, and Jill Crabtree, *How to Start a Respite Service for People with Alzheimer's and Their Families* (New York: Brookdale Foundation, 1987).

Richards, Marty. *Choosing a Nursing Home.* Seattle: University of Washington Press, 1988.

Shirk, Evelyn. *After the Stroke.* New York: Prometheus, 1995.

Skata, Ken. *American Guidance for Seniors.* San Luis Obispo, CA: Impact, 1995.

Task Force on Aging, Church Council of Greater Seattle. *How to Hire Helpers.* Seattle: Church Council of Greater Seattle, 1989.

———. *Reclaiming Time.* Seattle: Church Council of Greater Seattle, 1989.

Walker, Susan. *Keeping Active.* San Luis Obispo, CA: Impact, 1995. (A guide to activities and resources to keep seniors active and involved across generations.)

PART V
Planning for Wellness and Renewal

10
Staying Well and Keeping Fit

*Build today, then strong and sure,
with a firm and ample base;
ascending and secure,
shall tomorrow find its place.*
—Henry Longfellow, "The Builder"

Everyone wants to be well and fit as a foundation for a quality life. Self-care means nurturing the essentials of wellness—a deep sense of well-being, freedom from pain, energizing goals, and a renewing lifestyle. Since life renewal is the centerpiece of self-care, we will focus on ways that caregivers can renew themselves. In a fast-changing world, caregivers are forced by events to "re-new" themselves continually.

Another motive for maintaining a wellness and fitness program is to be in optimal condition for arduous care tasks. We assume that you know the rules for maintaining optimal health; but if you need a refresher, look up the *Wellness Made Easy* program.[1]

Wellness for Caregivers

Wellness is a state of well being that goes beyond good mental and physical health. Wellness means that you

- determine that the quality of your life is satisfying;
- follow the rules of good health and prevent unhealthful conditions from entering your daily life;

- maintain a buoyant and optimistic attitude;
- perceive yourself as happy and live each day to the fullest;
- view your life as fairly free of painful chronic illness; and
- possess a drive toward wellness (sometimes called a *will to wellness,* which is similar to the will to live—that strong desire to live a long and healthy life).

We will explore these various dimensions of caregiver wellness from research and opinions of experts. Many of the suggestions are adapted from *Healthy People: 2000*[2] and the surgeon general's report on health promotion and disease prevention in America.[3]

Your Lifestyle and Wellness

Are you promoting wellness in your own lifestyle? The following list of positive activities that reflect a healthful lifestyle has been gleaned from the previous chapters.

- You know and follow a healthful diet. This includes supplements that strengthen your immune system.
- You have an exercise program that is satisfying and meets wellness standards.
- You have a carefully monitored rest and relaxation routine.
- You adapt easily to changes and disappointments in your life.
- You have periodic outbursts of joy and happiness.
- You have many positive expectations and view most life events positively.
- You view everyday stressors as a challenge, and you experience satisfaction in meeting them.

- You are part of a support network.
- You identify and communicate feelings easily.
- You look for opportunities to express your gratitude and generosity.
- You have a sense of humor.
- You have a satisfactory spiritual outlook on life.
- You keep your hostility on a short leash (remember your heart when someone cuts you off in traffic, for example).
- You have checked your home for safety hazards—accidents, fire, disaster preparation, radiation, carcinogenic chemicals.
- You protect your sight and hearing from environmental damage.
- You use alcohol sparingly, if at all, and are cautious in using prescription drugs.
- You have regular health checkups and immunizations.
- You maintain your mental health through an active, socially involved life.
- You are involved in service to others and realize the self-enhancing benefits of service.
- You avoid smoking.
- You control your weight.

This is a long starter list. You can add more items that describe your ideas of wellness. While your attention is focused on wellness, we suggest that you check the items in the preceding list that you are meeting satisfactorily. Underline those items that you want to work on for the lifestyle planning activity later in this chapter.

Your care receiver can profit from promoting well-being also. If his or her well-being is enhanced, your care burden will be reduced. Betty Friedan surveyed attitudes toward well-being in older adults.[4] She reported that a positive attitude and an adventurous approach to life were the keys to living well. Similarly, Betty Alderson's survey of attitudes about well-being revealed that a sense of humor was especially useful to regain well-being when things went wrong or when the older adults could not seem to do anything about their problems.[5]

Happiness: A Part of Wellness

From Ancient Greece through modern times, happiness was regarded as a virtuous state and a goal of life. The Declaration of Independence includes the phrase "pursuit of happiness" as a human right. There are abundant reminders in everyday life that not many people are happy, meaning that they do not experience a sense of well-being over time, have few pleasures, and possess little joy in their lives. As a caregiver, you know that there is little happiness flowing from the care of a very ill person. The sadness and vicarious pain that are experienced often override the satisfaction of giving service. The goal for such service is more a feeling of well-being and satisfaction from the process of doing something socially significant or performing a needed personal service. The emphasis here is on **doing.** If you act in ways that make you feel good, you will be happy.

Jocelyn said, "After my mother died, I could see from this perspective that all I did for her has returned as a gift. I feel calm and peaceful now, and happy that I had come to know her well during this trying time." Jocelyn's reaction illustrates how life satisfactions and happiness, to a large extent, are a consequence of the positive way events are perceived, not the way things actually exist. You probably have acquaintances, for example, who seem to have everything—security, family, status, health, talent, and achievements—but appear to be desperately unhappy. You probably have discovered also that happiness is an inner state of being and is not contingent on outside events, possessions, or conditions of life.

The Good and Bad News about Happiness

While the popular belief is true that the more good conditions in life a person experiences, the happier that person becomes. Such things as status, income, toys, health, meaning, education, success, freedom, active lifestyle, and enjoyment are a few such conditions that spell happiness. The bad news, however, is that these good things are not evenly distributed in the population. There are *haves* and *have-nots* that erode the happiness myth. What are your beliefs about happiness?

The good news is that there are some personal traits that help people rise above deprivation from the good things of life. The main attitude, as we said, is that it is not what you **have** that makes you happy, but the **way you view life** in your unique setting.

There are some characteristics of happy people that Michael Fordyce has found form his own and others' studies of happy people. If you want to be happy, check these prerequisites:

- Be active and keep busy.
- Plan time for socializing.
- Do meaningful, productive work.
- Be organized and plan well.
- Avoid worry.
- Lower expectations.
- Think positive, optimistic thoughts.
- Orient life to the present.
- Work on being healthy.
- Develop an outgoing personality.
- Be yourself.

- Remove negative feelings.
- Maintain some close relationships.
- Think about what you could do to be happier.[6]

Application Activities

- Check those characteristics of happy people on the previous list that describe you now.
- Put an X in front of those characteristics you want to include in your renewal plans later.

One self-help suggestion for increasing your sense of well being is to conduct a *positive memory harvest*. This activity would be useful especially after a long dry spell of little or no pleasure. This is a simple effort to recall pleasant events in your earlier life. Follow these steps:

1. Seat yourself in a comfortable chair. Close your eyes. Relax your muscles, using your favorite relaxation procedure.
2. After about two minutes of relaxation go back a few years; quickly scan those years and focus on three or four happy events that took place. Visualize the pleasant activities, the people who were meaningful to you, the feelings you had—pleasure, joy, satisfaction. These would be times when you feel especially good about yourself, too, such as when you were creating music, art, or poetry, participating in a sports event, having Grandmother read to you, enjoying family picnics, and holiday singing, to name a few starter examples. Scrupulously avoid focusing on unpleasant events that made you feel sad, inadequate, uncomfortable, or frustrated.

3. Pick one or two of the pleasant events and mull them over for a few minutes, enjoying the good feelings these memories evoke in the present.
4. Open your eyes and focus back on your present situation, fully awake. Stretch and keep the good feelings you just recalled firmly in your awareness.
5. Tell yourself that you can be happy now, too, and that you can make your own happiness.

Family Environment and Well-Being

Well-being depends upon your ability to assess the presence of environmental danger and to be able to use this information to avoid harm. For example, you may look at your care environment positively. You observe that you have a friendly and helpful family, as well as a cooperative and congenial care receiver. You may also look at yourself as a competent person in command of the care scene.

With the positive conditions described here, you probably would experience a sense of well-being and good health. Conversely, you might have all the desirable personal traits, but you assessed your family environment as hostile and your care recipient as uncooperative, surly, and demanding. You would feel frustrated and demeaned. Yet you would survive adequately because of your self-care skills, your personal strengths, and awareness of the positives in your care situation.

If your care environment is unsavory and unsupportive, however, it would undoubtedly reduce your sense of well-being. Your choices at least are clear. You could work harder on changing family attitudes; you could insulate yourself against the negative reactions of your care receiver, or you could hope that your traits of confidence, personal power, and stress tolerance would sustain you enough to experience some sense of well-being.

Vulnerability to Pain

The topic of pain probably is very close to you, as a caregiver. Since most caregivers are middle-aged or older, they are more vulnerable to pain from chronic conditions than a younger person would be. You probably have all the aches and pains that go with normal aging. So, your self-care program could include management of these normal, physical, psychological, and spiritual pains.

Severe and chronic pain, however, is an enemy of well-being and should be checked by your physician. Physical pain is considered chronic if it persists for more than eight weeks.[7] If you have experienced broken bones or surgery, for example, you can expect associated pain to last up to six weeks.

Managing Your Pain

Muscle problems are a common cause of chronic pain.[8] As you think of your pain management plan, consider employing one or more of the following strategies:

- As emotional stress leads to tense muscles, which eventually causes severe pain, look at muscular pain as a measure of tension rather than illness. This kind of pain may radiate to other parts of your body. The self-help relaxation program described in the earlier discussion on stress is one approach to treating this type of pain. Massage therapy is a great aid to muscle relaxation also.

- If you suffer from a form of arthritis, include in your wellness plan a treatment program from a rheumatologist to control your arthritic pain. Stiff muscles and painful joints related to overuse or degenerative conditions are a key source of acute and chronic pain in older adults. Chronic conditions such as rheumatoid arthritis and osteoarthritis can be especially severe and limiting. They can rob you of an active life, even curtailing short walks
- As spasms and cramps are extremely painful and could be related to muscle misuse or overuse, if they persist have them checked out by a sports medicine specialist.
- As postural problems from weak muscles, imbalance, or hereditary weaknesses are sources of chronic pain, utilize treatments from a qualified physical therapist to ease these problems.
- Have internal chronic pain checked carefully by an internist to detect serious illness early.
- Attend to what your body is telling you with the pain. Consider the possibility that your pain may be an expression of a difficult life problem. For example, are you carrying your caregiving burdens on your back? If you have exhausted the medical search for causes and treatments of your internal pain, you may want to consult a psychologist who specializes in treating chronic pain with psychological methods.
- Focus on some other topic during the pain. If you worry or obsess about the pain, it may get worse.
- Carry on your daily routines, even if they are uncomfortable.
- Begin a moderate exercise program. Keep in mind that an activity that is too strenuous may make the pain worse. Walking, ski machines, stationary bicycles, and swimming are good activities to work through the pain with minimum risk. Give yourself

an *I can do* message to help you over the initial resistance and lagging motivation to continue.
- Pay special attention to chronic back pain. Caregivers are vulnerable, with their heavy lifting and reaching tasks. Problems arise also from postural defects, excessive weight, standing or sitting for long periods, cramped sleeping positions, congenital back problems, excessive or inappropriate lifting, high heels, weak abdominal muscles, and some unknown causes, to name a few. Psychological stress complicates back problems also. Do not be misled by the fact that painful backs are such a common problem among caregivers, and do not take the symptoms lightly. It would be prudent to check out the first sign of pain with an orthopedic specialist, as well as go over the preceding checklist of causes, in order to correct as many as possible with self-help.

Psychological and Spiritual Sources of Pain

Physical pain has its counterparts in psychological pain and spiritual suffering. Caregivers occasionally suffer pain that does not have a name. It is experienced as a deep ache or persistent longing for relief. This pain is associated with intense sadness or deep depression. Sometimes it is experienced in the form of agonizing despair, intense loneliness, or longing for another, happier time. Occasionally, this pain manifests itself in the form of debilitating self-reproach or self-pity.

Often reminders of humiliating failures send caregivers into despondency or feelings of emptiness. There are many more unnamed sufferings that afflict us. Some show up in our bodies in the form of an aching heart, a tight stomach, cramped bowels, shortness of breath, loss of appetite, or anxious hand wringing.

Coping with Psychic Pain

The big question is: What can a caregiver who is experiencing this kind of suffering do about it? In addition to our suggestions for coping and utilizing inner resources, you can ask yourself in the spirit of self-care: *What is the meaning of this suffering? What can I learn from this experience? How much of this suffering can I accept as a given part of living? How much of my present pain is related to my caregiving role? How much can be attributed to my long-standing personal problems and personality traits? How can I relate this painful experience to my family, and how will they take it? Where can I find comfort and reassurance? What can I do for myself to find courage, strength, and renewed commitment?*

We hope that contemplation of the preceding questions and applying the substance of this book will provide some insight, comfort, and courage to go on. With severe or prolonged pain and suffering, however, be willing to seek help from those spiritual counselors, secular psychotherapists, and primary care physicians you have come to know and trust.

Lifestyle Renewal

Renewal means to "make new again." Renewal is an important self-care goal, especially if you are one of those caregivers who feels "trapped on a treadmill." Perhaps a "prison" and "going to seed" might be more apt metaphors to describe your caregiving setting. What image comes to mind as you reflect on your current care situation? When your life begins to feel dull, boring, and lifeless, it is time to consider a renewal strategy and construct some new images.

This renewal effort should be undertaken when you are not in crisis, in the throes of change, or burning out. These extreme circumstances require a comprehensive coping strategy. After the crisis is over, your renewal program focused on achieving life satisfaction, enjoyment, and task efficiency can be undertaken.

Your Strategy for Renewal

Renewal strategy requires new goals for self-improvement. It is based on the premise that we must keep learning throughout our lives. You would be amazed at how much you have learned about yourself and about life over the years. We learn from our failures as well as from our successes. We learn from suffering, loving, and risking. We suggest that after each life event you ask, *What is this experience trying to teach me?* Then move on with new goals and plans.

You learn also that no matter how hard you try to please, not everyone will love you. You learn that commitment is important to relationships. You learn how to pace yourself and to conserve energy. You learn how you affect others positively and negatively. You learn that self-pity, guilt, resentment, and bitterness are poisonous. You learn the rewards of service. The most important learning is that life is an endless process of self-discovery. Renewal is a strategy to increase and perpetuate that self-discovery learning.

Goals for Your Renewal Plans

Simple renewal plans include setting specific goals for enriching your life or for improving your caregiving skills.

For example, you may want to reconstitute your piano-playing skill and spend more time listening to your favorite music. During these past months, caregiving has eaten up all your time, and you are beginning to feel dull and listless. Playing the piano again and taking time to listen to music is in the renewal spirit and is something that can be done at home without taking precious respite time.

In another example, a caregiver wants to launch an entirely new creative activity—watercolor. She wants to take a watercolor class at the local community college.

A third example of a renewal plan includes a community service project. This caregiver wants to volunteer at the local food bank during her six hours of respite time each week. She felt that serving people other than herself and her care receiver would energize her again.

The last two examples are modest and realistic goals for caregivers who can manage only a few hours of respite a week. The potential of enrichment goals is endless.

At the level of caregiving skill you may want to consider a professional renewal effort also. Examples of goals would be increasing communication effectiveness with your care receiver, improving stress management skills, and finding a dependable respite resource.

You may also want to examine your present lifestyle with the goal of making changes. Examples would be doing more exercises, eating low-fat meals, and getting more rest. The next section includes specific methods for planning your life renewal. This renewal process is a lifelong effort, especially in times of rapid change.

Your Renewal Plans

Self-enrichment. What are your wishes, dreams, and aspirations for enriching your life?

- *Step 1.* List your wishes here.
- *Step 2.* Change your wishes to goals.
- *Step 3.* Select one goal to work on now.
- *Step 4.* Develop a plan to reach that goal—cite resources needed, people involved, and timetables required.

Professional renewal. Use the same steps for developing your professional caregiving renewal plan. What are your wishes and hopes for renewing of your caregiving responsibilities?

- *Step 1.* Decide what skills you want to improve.
- *Step 2.* Change your hopes and desires for professional development into goals.
- *Step 3.* Decide which goal is most important now.
- *Step 4.* Develop a plan to realize your top professional renewal goal.

Examples are (1) making a self-care contract (Appendix A), and (2) improving communication with your recipient. You have noted, for instance, that Dad's dementia is getting worse. He does not pay attention to you anymore, but you would like more meaningful discussions with him. Your plan could include making clear statements of what you want from him, listening to his reactions to your requests, and looking for clear indications from his behavior that your message is getting through (nods, smiles, vocalizations, head shaking, etc.) Included in your plan would be a target date for noting improvements, such as one week. You would be alert to his increased interest when you pay close attention to his stories, complaints, requests, or ravings. You would also have in your plan the study of communication problems with particular patients, such as those with Alzheimer's disease. You would also practice making clear "I" statements when you make requests of him, such as, "I want you to take a shower before supper tonight." These requests are stated assertively, positively, and directly to the point. It is clear to him that this is an important personal request from you.

Do not give up. If one communication approach does not work well, then try another. You will know when you have found a winner because your energy, pleasure, and motivation levels will soar. Finally, find ways to reward this increased communication to keep it going, but without sounding patronizing. Do not forget to reward yourself also.

Developing a Fitness Program

Let us assume you want to be more physically fit. You set some goals to increase your strength and endurance. You know all about the benefits. You have the motivation to act. Now you need a plan of action. Write your answers to the following questions:

1. What are some activities you enjoy, such as walking and bicycling?
2. Where will you do them?
3. When can you fit them into your schedule?
4. How much time will you spend each day?
5. Who will support and encourage you?
6. What obstacles do you foresee that will sabotage your good intentions and efforts?

Additional Sources of Renewal Goals

As you read the previous chapters you probably noted some skills or attitudes you wanted to acquire. You might start with dealing with the essentials for caregiver survival listed in the introduction. Try completing the following:

- My burnout prevention and coping goals and plans are—.
- The survivor qualities I want and plan to acquire are—.
- Stress management skills I need and plan to acquire are—.
- Skills for changing self-defeating thinking and plans for changing them include—.
- My goals and plans for improving my support network are—.
- I want to fulfill my needs for intimacy and plan to do so by—.
- I want to strengthen my spiritual life by—.
- I want to develop a sharper sense of humor by—.
- I wish to expand my cultural awareness by doing the following—.
- My plan for my life after caregiving includes—.
- I want to cope better with my feelings of depression and despair by—.
- My anger and guilt control plans include—.
- My worry and pain control plans are—.
- I want to improve my communication and helping skills by—.
- My plans for wellness, fitness, and well-being include—.
- I want to write my life story and my plan to do it is—.

Life after Caregiving

The average length of a stint of caregiving is five years.[9] What is your life going to be like after this intensive investment of time and energy? Assuming that you have survived your caregiving time without damage to your body, psyche, and/or spirit, you can anticipate better times to come. In the future, as you look back you will be able to extract from your caregiving experience the strengths you acquired, the skills you learned, and the trust you developed in yourself and powers outside yourself—be they God, family, friends, church, health workers, or support groups.

When death comes to your patient you will naturally mourn this event. You will also very likely experience relief now that your caregiving tasks are finished and the future is open. Your patient's death is not the end of meaning and hope in your life unless you choose despair and self-pity.

Future avenues of growth and pleasure that you might wish to explore are:

- Travel (day trips or extended cruises and excursions).
- Volunteering (a good way to meet new friends).
- Joining an interest group.
- Sharing your gifts (sewing, music, visiting shut-ins).
- Writing your life story.
- Entertaining and practicing hospitality in your groups.
- Learning computers and surfing the Internet.
- Visiting friends and renewing old acquaintances.
- Finding a part-time job that intrigues you.

If you are thinking of a full-time job or a new career, your caregiving experience has career potential. If you found that care of your patient was rewarding or that you now need income, you might find an attractive career in the growing field of assisted living. Corporations that specialize in assisted living services to primary caregivers in their own homes or in group-home settings are looking for experienced people like you.

On the other hand, you may just want to sit and enjoy your new freedom for a while without feeling pressured to *do something constructive*. You will have many choices.

Life Review

Some caregivers carry an image of being on a treadmill or a carousel. They mean that their life goes on monotonously round and round each day—that their life does not seem to be going anywhere. Have you felt this way about your caregiving period of life? Whether or not this image is a problem for you, we suggest that you set a long-term goal to write your life story.

Good Things about Writing Your Story

The usefulness of this activity is that it has a validating effect on your life. You realize that your life has had meaning, and you now see problems and events, including your present caregiving role, in perspective. If you focus on your strengths and talents (and everyone has some) as they evolve, you will very likely experience a surge of self-pride and sense of achievement. You would do well to minimize your mistakes, limitations, and humiliations. You might find it more difficult to write about your strengths and achievements than your limitations and failures, since early cultural conditioning emphasized self-effacement rather than self-assertion. We suggest that you describe your more rewarding experiences and perceptions of your strengths.

How to Write Your Life Story

Write in your own style. As a starter, you can use an image like a book chapter, a life journey, or seasons to describe your life. You could begin with the present and work back or start with childhood and move forward by stages of development. You could do a narrative to the present combined with a journal of your present feelings and experiences as a caregiver.

At first glance, such a project probably seems daunting. Writing your life story is a lifelong project, but you can start now. It will be healing for you, and your family will be grateful for your story. You will find insights and learnings cropping up unexpectedly. Make a special note of these side trips to ponder later. You will find that as you continue this project into your later years, it will be quite therapeutic. Writing life reviews is a prescriptive activity for older folks to validate their lives, give them a feeling of closure, and view their life events in historical perspective.

Getting Started

The big problem is to get going. We suggest that you describe a few family anecdotes. Later you can provide the contexts and transitions. Another suggestion is to collect photos, clippings, and favorite poems that tell a story by themselves. You can just add some descriptive material about who, when, where, and what. Add your own poems, letters, and articles.

Once started, the excitement and energy of the writing itself will sustain your motivation to go on. One of the authors of this book, Marian, compiled a set of binders about her husband's long professional career, which kept him interested for hours during his last months of illness. It contained a chronology of pictures, letters, and clippings. The books were a great aid to help him recapture the pleasant memories of his long career; it also served as a treasured memorial for his family.

You might encourage your care receiver, if the person has the capacity, to write his or her life story also. Since writing is likely to be problematic, speaking to a tape recorder is a good alternative. Increased interest in life could be a side effect of your care receiver telling his or her story.

Putting It All Together

Wellness and fitness are essential for your survival and effective pain management. Self-renewal and self-enrichment, however, add those extra touches of life satisfaction and well-being that make it all worthwhile.

Renewal activities not only allow the burden of caregiving to be more tolerable but also add energy, instill hope, and generate enthusiasm for your caregiving tasks. The end products are a fulfilled and happy caregiver and a satisfied, well-cared-for recipient.

Notes

1. *Wellness Made Easy,* University of California, Berkeley, Wellness Letter (Berkeley, CA: Berkeley Wellness Letters, 1990).
2. *Healthy People: 2000.,* Publication no. 79-5071 (Washington, DC: U.S. Department of Health, Education, and Welfare, 1979).
3. Richard Winett, "A Framework for Health Promotion and Disease Prevention Programs," *American Psychologist* 50 (May 1995): 341–50.
4. Betty Friedan, *Fountain of Age* (New York: Simon and Schuster, 1993). (She emphasizes the importance of having a positive and adventurous stance toward life.)
5. Betty Alderson, "How Men and Women Cope with the Ups and Downs of Aging," *Remedy,* January/February 1995.

6. Michael Fordyce. *The Psychology of Happiness* (Fort Myers, FL: Cypress Lake Media, 1981).(A research-based approach to happiness.)
7. Norman Marcus, M.D., "How to Win the Chronic Pain Wars," *Bottom Line,* February 15, 1981, pp. 9–10.
8. Ibid.
9. Health Advisory Services, AARP, *A National Survey of Caregivers* (Washington, DC: American Association of Retired Persons, 1988).

Recommended References

Campbell, David. *If You Don't Know Where You're Going, You'll Probably End Up Somewhere.* Niles, IL: Argus Communications, 1974.

Church Council of Greater Seattle. *Reclaiming Time: Caregiver Relief and Renewal.* Seattle, WA: Church Council of Greater Seattle, 1995.

Gardner, John. *Self-Renewal.* New York: Harper, 1965.

Ory, Marcia, Ronald Abeles, and Paula Lipman. *Aging, Health and Behavior.* New York: Sage, 1991.

Appendixes

Appendix A
Making a Self-Care Contract

I PROMISE TO:

- be more aware of and honor my physical needs and my feeling experiences—listen to my body messages;
- be gentle, loving, and forgiving with myself;
- accept and celebrate my strengths;
- acknowledge and live with my limitations;
- accept help when offered—I will not try to do it all by myself;
- strengthen my support networks;
- strengthen my coping skills;
- share my grief and my joy more often;
- regularly seek respite care and other needed help;
- follow the self-care, wellness, and renewal guidelines of this book;
- set priorities for my highest good;
- live life to the fullest;
- identify situations that will have the greatest positive impact for me and avoid situations that will retard or destroy the impact (as in alcoholism, drug use, workaholism, and self-pity);
- insist that immediate family members be involved in direct care, and most certainly in equitable financial contributions;
- protect my freedom by not acquiescing to the inequitable or unreasonable requests and expectations of family members;

- feel good about myself for confronting family about shared responsibility;
- facilitate a family council meeting to consider issues of shared care, wills, trusts, respite plans, and funeral arrangements if death is imminent;
- learn to live comfortably with the contradiction that I want to give the best care I can and to make my care receiver feel comforted, valued, and esteemed, yet I must realize that these good-care efforts build dependency and generate more requests for service and attention and provoke greater feelings of helplessness; and try to empower the person in my care to do more for him- or herself.

Signed_____Date_____

Appendix B
Internet Web Sites for Caregivers*

- Start your search here / All in One—**http://www.albany.net/allinone/**
- Start your search here / Alta Vista—**http://altavista.digital.com/**
- Start your search here / Yahoo—**http://yahoo.com/**
- AIDS Information from NIH—**gopher://odie.niaid.nih.gov/11/aids**
- American Academy of Pediatrics—**http://www.aap.org/**
- American Cancer Society—**http://www.cancer.org/**
- American Diabetes Association—**http://www.diabetes.org/**
- American Heart Association—**http://www.amhrt.org/**
- American Medical Association—**http://www.amaassn.org/**
- Arthritis Foundation—**http://www.arthritis.org/**
- Back Pain Information—**http://www.sechrest.com/mmg/back/backpain.html/**
- Breast Cancer Information—**http://nysernet.org/bcic/**
- Centers for Disease Control—**http://www.cdc.gov/**

---

*Reproduced with permission of Bill Crounse, M.D., Vice President, Chief Information Officer, Overlake Hospital Medical Center, Bellevue, WA.

- CNN Health Interactive—**http: //www.cnn.com/index.html**
- Crohn's & Colitis Foundation—**http: //www.ccfa.org/**
- Depression Self-Test—**http: //www.med.nyu.edu/psych/screens/depres.html**
- Food and Drug Administration—**http: //www.fda.gov/**
- Health Answers—**http: //www.healthanswers.com/**
- Healthfinder—**http: //www.healthfinder.gov**
- Healthfront—**http: //healthfront.com/**
- Healthgate—**http: //www.healthgate.com/HealthGate/home.html**
- Healthgate Free Medline—**http: //www.healthgate.com/HealthGate/Medline/search**
- Heart Web—**http: //webasix.com/heartweb**
- Heart Point—**http: //www.heartpoint.com**
- Internet Health Forum—**http: //www.comed.com/index.spml**
- Medical Matrix—**http: //www.medmatrix.org/**
- Medicine Net—**http: //www.medicinenet.com/**
- Men's Fitness—**http: //www.mensfitness.com/**
- Men's Health—**http: //medic.med.uth.tmc.edu/ptnt/00000391.htm**
- Multimedia Medical Library—**http: //www.mmrl.com/medilibrary/**
- National Cancer Institute, CancerNet—**http: //wwwicic.nic.nih.gov/**
- National Health Information Center—**http: //nhicnt.health.org/**
- National Institutes of Health—**http: //www.nih.gov/**
- National Library of Medicine—**http: //www.nlm.nih.gov/**

- National Mental Health Association—**http: //www.worldcorp.com/dc-online/nhma/**
- National Stroke Association—**http: //www.stroke.org/**
- Netwellness Home Page—**http: //www.netwellness.org/**
- New Atlantis Healthcity—**http: //www.healthcity.com/**
- New England Journal of Medicine—**http: //www.nejm.org/**
- NIH Consensus on Impotence—**http: //test.nlm.nih.gov/nih/cdc/www/91txt.html**
- No Scalpel Vasectomy—**http: //www.noscalpelvasectomy.org/**
- Oncolink Cancer Information—**http: //oncolink.upenn.edu/**
- Overlake Hospital Medical Center—**http: //www.overlakehospital.org/**
- Pregnancy, Ovulation & Childbirth Calculator—**http: //www.olen.com/baby**
- Prostate Cancer Infolink—**http: //www.comed.com/Prostate/Introduction.html**
- Travel Health Information—**http: //www.intmed.mcw.edu/ITC/Health.html**
- University of Washington—**http: //www.hslib.washington.edu/**
- Wellness Interactive Network—**http: //www.stayhealthy.com**
- Your First Health Risk Appraisal—**http: //www.youfirst.com**

With its low cost and global reach, the Web is a bonanza for unscrupulous purveyors of "snake oil." When it comes to something as important as your health, how can you be sure the medical information you are getting can be trusted? Here are some tips:

- **Who is providing the information?** Trust established government sources, academic medical centers, named and known medical institutions, not-for-profit organizations, and other sources that clearly list their identity, credentials, and qualifications.
- **Is the information current?** The best sites will not only clearly identify who is responsible for the information provided but will also tell you when it was posted.
- **Is someone trying to sell you something?** Take extra caution with sites whose primary purpose is to sell you medical goods or services. If it sounds too good to be true . . . it probably is.

Appendix C
Caregiver Survey

I would appreciate your frank and complete answers to the following general questions. Your answers will not be connected with your name to maintain strict confidentiality. The information will be used to support illustrative points in our forthcoming book. Our basic assumption is that being a caregiver, or having gone through the experience, you are a first-hand authority on the subject. Feel free not to answer a question if it appears too intrusive or painful. Thanks very much for your help in making this guide for caregivers more useful.

Please tell me briefly what your caregiving situation is, or has been.

What are, or have been, the most distressing aspects of your caregiving experience?

How did you experience this distress (your feelings, sensations, thoughts)?

What have been the rewarding aspects of your caregiving experience?

What did you do to ease your distress?
    What inner resources did you draw upon to ease your burden?

What would you say are your greatest strengths as a caregiver?

What greater personal resources would you have wanted?

Did you seek outside help? If so, what kind? How was it helpful, not helpful, or hindering?

Which organizations or professionals supported you most during your caregiving time? What kinds of support did they offer?

Did you receive help from friends and relatives? What types of help were received and how effective was their help?

Were any personal problems (including physical health), apart from caregiving pressures, making your caregiving more difficult?

What are your most effective methods of coping with stressors of caregiving?

Is there anything else you would like to add about your caregiver experience?

Thank you very much for your assistance on this project.